SLEEPING APART NOT FALLING APART

. . . .

To my husband Fraser — I couldn't have written this book without you

SLEEPING APART NOT FALLING APART

How to get a good night's sleep *and* keep your relationship alive

JENNIFER ADAMS

FINCH PUBLISHING
SYDNEY

Sleeping Apart Not Falling Apart

First published in 2013 in Australia and New Zealand by Finch Publishing Pty Limited, ABN 49 057 285 248, Suite 2207, 4 Daydream Street, Warriewood, NSW, 2102, Australia.

13 8 7 6 5 4 3 2

Copyright © 2013 Jennifer Adams

The author asserts her moral rights in this work throughout the world without waiver. All rights reserved. No part of this publication may be reproduced, stored in a retrieval system or transmitted in any form or by any means (electronic or mechanical, through reprography, digital transmission, recording or otherwise) without the prior written permission of the publisher.

There is a National Library of Australia Cataloguing-in-Publication entry available at the National Library.

Edited by Laura Russell
Editorial assistance by Megan Drinan
Text typeset in ITC Legacy Serif by Pier Vido
Cover design by Ingrid Kwong
Printed by Griffin Press

The information on page 149 from Dr Barbara Bartlik is reproduced with permission from Bottomline Publications website. Copyright © 2012 by Boardroom Inc., www.BottomLinePublications.com

Reproduction and Communication for educational purposes
The Australian Copyright Act 1968 (the Act) allows a maximum of one chapter or 10% of the pages of this work, whichever is the greater, to be reproduced and/or communicated by any educational institution for its educational purposes provided that the educational institution (or the body that administers it) has given a remuneration notice to Copyright Agency Limited (CAL) under the Act. For details of the CAL licence for educational institutions contact: info@copyright.com.au

Finch titles can be viewed and purchased at www.finch.com.au

Contents

Prologue: My bedtime story   vii

Introduction: Setting the scene   1

1: A social history of sleep   4

2: The science of sleep   19

3: The truth about bed sharing   37

4: The decision   71

5: Negotiating the outcome   107

6: How to make sleeping separately work   126

7: What will the neighbours think?   168

8: Night, night, sleep tight   196

Author's note

As I was writing this book, the thorny issue of using a gender neutral pronoun raised its ugly head. My solution was to use 'they' instead of 'he' or 'she'. While it can be argued that this is not technically or grammatically correct, it is a practice that is becoming more widely accepted in the face of there being no true, singular gender-neutral pronoun. My intent is that where 'they', 'them' or 'their' is used, readers will insert the gender pronoun appropriate for them.

PROLOGUE

My bedtime story

After marrying mid-2007, a number of people enquired as to how married life was treating me. I could happily reply each time that all was well. As my husband had moved into my house, those who knew me well enough would sometimes progress to asking how we were settling into a bedroom together – more specifically, how we were settling into my bedroom together. This was an easy answer.

No settling in required. We had separate bedrooms.

Over the next couple of years, I found myself caught up in discussions from time to time that would lead me to talk about 'our separate bedrooms'. While I had no concerns about sharing this aspect of my life (think 'heart' and 'sleeve' and you have me) I found there were many people who had similar arrangements, but dissimilar approaches to sharing this fact. I was intrigued as to why people were so secretive about, what was for me, a practical solution to the problem of not being able to sleep at night because of sleeping incompatibilities.

A common concern raised was that my marriage was either in some fairly serious and early trouble, or that my husband Fraser and I must be going through some growing pains and were sleeping apart while we worked these issues through. I knew my marriage wasn't on shaky ground at all and would always reassure the person enquiring that all was well.

From these early discussions, I developed an interest in people's perceptions of separate sleeping. My curiosity set me off on a mission to discuss the topic whenever the opportunity presented itself. What I found was an assortment of attitudes and honesty about the issue – and a recurring theme of reluctance to be open about the practice for fear of social judgement.

Those conversations, and the encouragement I received to share thoughts and opinions on the topic, resulted in this book. I think there are many couples, or individuals in couples, who would like to know there are others who need their sleep so badly that they prioritise it over and above the need to lie next to their partners at night. I also think that they would like to know there are other couples who sleep separately some nights or every night because of this need for sleep. And importantly, I think that knowing they are not alone in choosing to sleep separately would help them feel okay.

But back to the beginning. This is how I found myself in my own bed each night.

My path to marriage was a little delayed. I did not tie the knot until I was 41. In my early twenties and through to my mid-thirties, I had boyfriends with whom I very happily shared a bed. In fact, sharing a bed with a partner and snuggling into him to fall asleep was the fantasy I had read about in many a *Cleo* or *Cosmopolitan* magazine. I thoroughly enjoyed living out this fantasy at that stage of my life. I loved sleeping with my partners; the closeness of sharing a bed each night and sharing a space in a house or apartment that was ours. I didn't imagine this would ever change.

A two-year relationship at age 34 saw me sharing a bed with a new boyfriend – we'll call him Brent. However, after about six months I started to have issues with disturbed sleep. Not only did Brent's snoring bother me, but he liked to have the room at a rather chilly 19 degrees Celsius every night. This was fine in summer, but uncomfortably cold in winter. I don't care about science or logic – it seemed colder in winter!

As our relationship progressed, Brent became increasingly upset if he was woken when I went to bed after him. This happened frequently as I tended to go to bed later than him more often than not. The situation created a tangible tension—but in the spirit of trying harder to make the relationship work, I tried to be as invisible as possible and silently prepared to glide into bed every night. This is never an easy task when you are using an ensuite bathroom for bedtime preparation.

After trying to manage in these sleeping conditions for about 18 months, I endured three nights of practically no sleep due to Brent's snoring and a 'clicking' air conditioner. The anxiety caused by being scared to wake him didn't help either. The sleeplessness was so bad that even after sneaking off to another room I lay awake, overcome by waves of adrenalin caused by the stress of not sleeping. The situation became so dire that I saw my doctor who prescribed sleeping tablets for the first time in my life. This was a low point as I began to ponder a future of either sleepless nights or repeat prescriptions.

(I do realise that there are people, such as mothers of young babies, who may think that three nights of sleeplessness is a bit lightweight and not much to complain about. I have always admired those who can exist on little sleep, but my body's wiring is different and I struggle without at least seven hours sleep.)

Faced with this ongoing dilemma, I started to sneak out more often to the spare room. However, Brent did not approve and saw it as an unnecessary overreaction on my part. His solution was that I should sleep with earplugs every night. His interpretation of a traditional relationship involved sharing a bed every night even if it meant that my comfort, my much-needed nightly rest and my health were suffering. My attempts to talk about the issue were met with much tongue clicking and dismissive annoyance and comments that 'lots of women deal with a snoring partner' so really, I should just get over it. I won't even start to describe the conversations about the air conditioner and room temperature.

As it happened, I couldn't 'just get over it'. As each night appraoched, I became increasingly stressed and anxious that I wouldn't get enough sleep to function the next day. Much to my dismay, going to bed started to become a stressful event.

A combination of factors (including the sleep issues) brought about the demise of the relationship. The ending, while sad, was also tinged with joy at the prospect of being free from the nightly trauma of sharing a bed with Brent. I returned to live in my house and oh so happily began sleeping in my own bed again. The calm I felt, knowing there would be no snoring, no air conditioner wheezing and clicking and no recriminations for not being able to sleep was indescribable. The freedom of choosing when and under what conditions I slept had never felt so welcome and important.

Then I met my husband. The throes of an early relationship mask many practical ills. The first nights Fraser and I spent in a bed together were filled with the activities of a new relationship – dinners out, a healthy amount of alcohol and the enthusiastic passion a couple enjoys. This combination would work well to help us sleep through the night.

Once we started to settle down into the comfortable rhythm of who was going to stay at whose place, I started to experience restless sleep again. When we slept over at each other's homes and I couldn't sleep, I would sneak off to the couch if we were at my house or the floor of the loungeroom at his place. This was not an ideal solution and did result in a less than satisfactory night's sleep and a little stress. However, as we weren't living together, the broken sleep was interspersed with regular, good sleep alone at my house.

An added complication is that Fraser is a tradesman. He needs to be up at 5 am most mornings, works hard all day, and then wants to be in bed by about 9 pm. He did very well to stay up later when we first started seeing each other, but not surprisingly, he couldn't sustain the late nights.

After about four months, Fraser and I decided that he should move into my house. The idea of sharing a bed was causing us both some consternation but we didn't have an honest conversation about this aspect of sharing a home. The standard practice is quite simple: when you move in with someone, you share a bed with them. So that's what we did. Fraser moved in, and we started sharing a bed. We lasted a week.

Fraser's snoring kept me awake and we didn't easily share the confines of a bed. As we were both in our late thirties, our ability to adapt to new situations was low, so the situation wasn't one that either of us could easily overlook. Not that we confessed this to one another immediately. However, we did eventually have a chat.

During the chat we agreed to only share a bed on the weekends as we needed to get our sleep during the week. That plan lasted about two weekends. A complicating factor to sharing a bed is that Fraser's snoring is not what I would describe as 'run-of-the-mill'. It is on another level entirely and in time we would find out that he has sleep apnoea.

So after three weeks of Fraser living in my house, we moved to sleeping in separate beds every night. I think secretly we were both relieved we had made the decision, but didn't share this relief with each other with too much enthusiasm for fear of hurting the other's feelings. We still enjoyed lying in each other's beds before we went to sleep or upon waking, having a kiss goodnight and a kiss good morning and dozing with each other in one bed, or the other, on the weekend.

This was how our set of rules evolved to manage the challenge of sleeping in separate rooms while still showing each other that we were committed to the relationship.

On a very practical level, it became evident over time that sharing a room would have been problematic. Fraser rises early most days and retires to bed early in the evening. In contrast, I am a night person. I will often stay up until 11 pm and beyond, and I do so love a lie-in on weekends. I am overly attached to reading in bed and doing this in a shared bed when your partner is already asleep is awkward and asking for trouble.

There would also have been issues with room temperature and bed coverings. Fraser can withstand quite a warm room in summer – I need a fan. Fraser sleeps with minimal bed clothes – I like many layers. Fraser doesn't mind getting into a cold bed in the winter – I can't live without an electric blanket. All of these added to a mounting list of bed incompatibilities and a realisation that separate rooms really was the best option for us. We both agreed that being resentful towards the other person because one of us had to give up the when and how of sleeping wouldn't have made for a healthy relationship. Coming to this realisation made us feel more confident in the decision to sleep separately.

I know that our decision is not for everyone. Many people I know wouldn't dream of not sharing a bed every night with their partner: they see a shared bed as an important part of their relationship. I believe our decision to sleep apart has solidified our relationship. As we spend every night apart, we are forced to be very honest with each other about our commitment to the relationship. The decision to have separate rooms meant that we retain a significant part of who we are as individuals and have to talk about what this means for us as a couple.

We take great care not to exclude each other from the part of our lives associated with a bedroom, as silly as that sounds. Lying around on each other's bed is commonplace and neither room is considered a private space that the other can't enter.

We have been together for nine years now, are very happy (notwithstanding the standard ups and downs any couple faces) and have a normal, functioning relationship. I often wonder if sleeping separately impacts on our relationship because we don't share the closeness of being in a bed together every night. When I weigh everything up though, I do wonder if we would still be together had it not been for our decision to have separate bedrooms. I guess we will never know. Of most importance is that our sleeping arrangements work for us - and we are the only people who really understand why and how it works.

As humans we tend to judge based on our own values and norms and this is why we condemn or criticise others who are different. Because their decision is not one that we would make, we often don't attempt to understand it.

So my sleeping story is not everyone's sleeping story. But I do know that there are thousands of couples whose sleeping story is similar to mine - and many thousands more who would like to at least try for themselves.

INTRODUCTION

Setting the scene

This book aims to provide interesting information and practical guidelines for those couples who face sleeping together with a degree of hesitation, are curious to find out if there are options they haven't thought of to solve their sleeping issues or want to know how other couples deal with the problem. The book may also prove useful to those couples who are struggling to make sleeping separately work by reviewing how they manage their current circumstances.

Sleeping apart can mean many things and take many forms – this book considers the range of behaviours sleeping separately may cover.

It is important to say up front that I support the many couples who sleep in the same bed night after night, spooning each other into blissful slumber, and waking happily next to each other ready to face the day. I certainly don't think that sleeping apart is for every couple, just as I don't think sleeping together is for everyone.

I also recognise that sleeping separately (especially in a separate room) is <u>not an option readily available to everyone</u>. Limited space, or particular domestic arrangements, may restrict the opportunity for one person to enjoy sleeping separately every night.

Where and how you sleep is only one aspect of a relationship and should assume an amount of importance that is right for each couple. As with every decision made in a partnership, all priorities need to be considered as part of a bigger picture. This includes respecting the other partner's needs as well as the needs of others in the equation such as children or extended family.

I researched widely to both back up and challenge my own thoughts about this topic. I had many, many conversations with people that I knew well and not so well. I also interviewed couples and individuals about their sleeping behaviours, both those who loved sleeping together and those who headed for separate rooms every night. I trawled the internet to pull together as much information as I could find from articles (academic, news-based and opinion pieces), forums, blogs and websites. I also found two books on the topic of the issues faced by couples sleeping together.

While writing the book I had an article published on Mia Freedman's *Mamamia* website in January 2011. The article elicited an enthusiastic response from readers and led to seven radio interviews across Australia. Comments and feedback from the article and the radio interviews are also used in the book.

All the formal and informal information gathered from these sources appears in different guises. Often after casual conversations I made notes of what was said and gained permission from each person to use their information. I found couples to interview through word-of-mouth, by asking readers of my blog to get in touch and by advertising on internet forums. I also sought permission from *mamamia.com.au* and Radio National's program *Life Matters* to use the comments in response to my article and interview, as well as from other sites and blogs that had content I wanted to use.

All names of people I interviewed or who submitted stories to me have been changed to respect each person's privacy. However, to give context to each story, I have included the age of the person as a minimum, and in most cases, their occupation and the amount of time they have been with their partner. While it was easier to find couples who were 40-plus and sleeping separately, the youngest couple I spoke with were 24 and 26 years old respectively.

I am so, so grateful to the many people who shared their personal details and stories. Some of the stories had me in stitches, while some had me feeling sympathy for the dire situations that people were in due to lack of sleep or a faltering relationship as a result of missing sleep.

1

A social history of sleep

'All this fuss about sleeping together. For physical pleasure I'd sooner go to my dentist any day.' – *Evelyn Waugh*

Sharing a bed with a partner is one of the cornerstones of a relationship. Or at least that's the message implied in contemporary Western culture. In the last few decades, our cultural practices seem to equate a successful relationship with successfully sharing a bed. It's an interesting logic. Recent research has found that 'social dictates as to how a person should sleep can easily result in a discrepancy between cultural sleep norms and an individual's biological needs'. Studies on the social aspects of sleep often reveal that 'sleep customs may not always be in the health interests of the individual'. But still, we keep jumping into bed with each other.

Socially accepted norms

A natural but complex process, sleep is a fundamental human need that, similar to the need to eat, has a social lens of judgement cast over it. This lens ascribes so much more to sleeping than its basic physiological function. While there is no judgement over the act of sleeping itself, when two people commit to a personal relationship there is an expectation that the couple will share a bed together each night to sleep. And while more couples than not are happy to walk this traditional path, why is sleeping apart so often frowned upon for couples? Why do so many people hide the fact that they are their own ideal sleeping partner? But most importantly, why do so many people endure sleepless night after sleepless night just to conform to a social norm?

Sleeping, in itself, is an individual activity. Ironically, many people choose to lie next to another person to do it. Gerhard Klösch, author of *Sleeping Better Together*, notes that 'sleep, as well as being a process, is also a behaviour evidenced by rituals associated with its onset and end'. And as we humans are wont to do, we like to share our behaviours and rituals with others. It's more fun that way.

Paul Rosenblatt, professor of family social science at the University of Minnesota and author of *Two in a Bed: The Social System of Couple Bed Sharing* writes about couples needing to learn to share a bed. Unfortunately, just as we can't all learn the mysteries of quantum physics, not everyone can learn to endure night after night of minimal or broken sleep simply for the sake of sharing a bed with the person they love – no matter how much fun those behaviours and rituals are.

Australian relationship expert and psychologist Jacqueline Saad says of sleeping apart, 'We find the idea strange as society has conditioned us to expect that a couple must share a bed. It signifies the sharing and joining of personal and spiritual space. There is a stigma attached to sleeping in separate beds which traditionally implies a breakdown in the relationship.'

Stephanie Coontz, a professor of history and family studies at Evergreen State College in Washington State argues that the weight of expectation on the marital bed is artificial and relatively new. She says that, 'It represents this cookie-cutter model that developed in the early 20th century that told people you had to get every single need met by this constant togetherness. It doesn't tie in with what we know about the variety of coupled relationships that have worked in history.' What's more, Coontz points out that the model doesn't fit contemporary life in which couples marry later, bringing more experiences and habits to their relationships.

The public face of sleep

As a culture that is heavily influenced by what we see in print and visual media, the portrayal of a couple sleeping 'together' has evolved from not showing couples together in bed at all, to the ubiquitous image of a married couple retiring to their twin beds (often clothed neck to ankle in flannelette) in many television shows and movies of the 1950s and 1960s, and finally to the point where couples, both hetero- and homosexual, are shown in a vast range of domestic arrangements, hopping into a bed together without anyone raising an eyebrow.

Apparently one of the ultimate TV trivia questions is: who was the first couple to be shown on television sleeping in the same bed? And it has different answers – depending on your definition of 'sleeping in the same bed'. According to most television trivia sources, *The Flintstones* (1960–6) holds the distinction of being the first television program to show a couple actually in bed together – albeit an animated couple. Other trivia buffs claim it was in a program titled *Mary Kay and Johnny*, first screened in America in 1947. Actors Mary Kay and Johnny Stearns starred in a television-based domestic comedy as a real-life couple living in a Greenwich Village apartment, and to keep production costs down, the show was filmed in the couple's real apartment, with their real bed.

However, there is contention as to whether Mary and Johnny were actually shown in the bed together, rather than showing their bedroom with just one bed, leading viewers to the conclusion that they both slept there. Another more popular show that featured a couple in bed was *I Love Lucy* in 1951.

Two episodes in the first year showed Lucy (Lucille Ball) and Ricky (Desi Arnez) in what appeared to be a king-size bed. But when they crawled under the sheets, and under their separate blankets, it was apparent there were two beds pushed together, each one made up separately. So technically they weren't in the same bed. In later episodes, once little Ricky was born, the beds were separated by a night stand. CBS suggested that the beds be pushed apart to diminish the impact of the suggested sexual history of Lucy and Ricky. Goodness knows how the viewers thought the child was conceived!

Indeed, whoever the first couple was, it is perhaps the pervasive image of domestic success involving a couple happily hopping into a bed every night and appearing rested and just as happy on waking the next morning that has helped to create the sought after image of night-time harmony to which we aspire. If you aren't blissfully slumbering next to your loved one, like they do on TV and in the movies, does that mean there's something wrong?

> *I suppose you see it on TV. For me, it started with* Bewitched. *The happy couple sleeps together and that's equated with marital bliss.*
> **Suzette, 40, administrative assistant, married 17 years**

> *Most couples on TV and in the movies always seem to get through a night's sleep without too much bother. They don't seem to be too troubled by their partner and often wake up with perfect hair and make-up. Maybe I'm generalising, but it isn't that way in my bedroom. Maybe I'm the one with the problem?*
> **Lulu, 42, legal professional, married 6 years**

But just as evolution continues on all fronts – we're challenged by constant social change whether we like it or not – the dynamics of the traditional relationship model are open to reinvention.

Pamela Smock, a University of Michigan sociologist says, 'Couples today are writing their own script, rewriting how to have a marriage.' She notes though, that husbands are less willing to change familiar patterns. 'Men are supposed to be one, dominant, and two, sexual,' she says. 'Their wives might be thrilled to have their own bedrooms, and see it as a romantic thing – going back to romance, going back to dating, to intimacy – but the husband might not see it that way. As a social pattern, this could increase. A lot of people I know fantasise about living in the same apartment building as their husband—but in a separate apartment. That could be next.'

> *I think it's a male ego thing that he wants me there. That's what it should be like and what we should do – according to him.*
> **Kaye, 66, married 14 years**

> *I know of males who insist that their wives sleep with them as they are the boss and are the dominant ones in the relationship. They think they have the right to say how things will be in their house.*
> **Matt, 47, senior manager, married 20 years**

A cultural shift in which more couples choose to sleep separately is reflected in statistics coming out of America. A survey by the National Sleep Foundation in 2001 found that 12 per cent of married Americans were sleeping alone; by 2005 this figure had grown to 23 per cent. Studies in England have found similar results with research in 2007 showing that more than a third of British couples frequently sleep in separate rooms. In 2009 *The New York Times* cited a survey of builders and architects which predicted that by 2015, 60 per cent of custom-built houses would have two master bedrooms. Gopal Ahluwalia, of America's National Association of Home Builders, observed that this was a 'market-driven demand that's going to continue'.

These statistics are not surprising when considered against the backdrop of cultural shifts that came out of social movements that gave women a louder voice and were focused on equality in male/female relationships. The traditional role of woman as homemaker and carer of the husband is no longer a given. All the stereotypes of a woman as a wife – including those in the bedroom – have been substantially challenged in recent decades.

> *This has never seemed to be a problem for us as we share both things. Chris baths the kids and does the vacuuming and still works pretty hard and I do too. Since we have three children, it's not a big thing for us to sleep in separate beds, separate rooms – it's just not a big issue.*
> Liz, 41, accountant, married 10 years

When did sleeping together become the norm?

Looking back on the sleeping habits of our predecessors, a couple sleeping in the same bed every night has not always been the norm. It is a modern construct and hasn't always been the 'cool thing to do'.

Cultural, historical influences have always played a part in determining contemporary social behaviours. Where and with whom you sleep is one of those behaviours. Klösch tells us that 'sleeping either in groups or in individual beds was the more common practice that researchers describe in humans from prehistoric societies to many contemporary non-European cultures' and that sleeping together is a 'sociocultural phenomenon, a fashion, and a lifestyle'.

Our cave-dwelling ancestors probably slept in groups for safety. This is still common practice in many tribal cultures when safety during sleep is needed (and possibly still in many houses around the world when those frightened by storms dash into another's bed for comfort). Many early civilisations adopted group sleep as a common practice because it was practical and afforded people a time and place to socialise. To address the issue of keeping the species alive, a common feature of group sleep was that a man and a woman would come together in a bed for procreation only – more than likely one that afforded some privacy. This practice is identified in writings on Greek and Egyptian cultural practices.

The evolution of the bed itself started to influence whether individuals were able to enjoy the luxury of sleeping alone. The availability of a bed and bedroom for oneself was initially reliant on wealth and social status – and in places such as Britain, definitely reliant on how big your castle was. If you had no wealth, social status or castle, you remained relegated to dorm-style sleeping facilities, or you might be lucky to have a pallet, trundle bed or bench in your lord's chamber. These conditions prevailed throughout the Middle Ages. The understanding from writings of those times is still the notion of group sleep as the norm with couples coming together in a private space for procreation only.

It wasn't until the late nineteenth century that regular bed sharing for couples became more common. The Industrial Revolution brought families from the country into towns and this move presented them with houses that were much smaller than the spacious country-style homes they had left. Therefore, sharing a bed shifted from being something a couple might do to enjoy some conjugal rights, to being a non-negotiable, night-time reality. But this didn't mean that everyone was happy with the arrangement.

Despite the growing practice of bed sharing, there were still social groups attached to the practice of sleeping separately. They did tend to be the wealthier members of society, who continued to uphold the notions of privacy and propriety found in a room of one's own.

Neil Stanley, a leading UK sleep research expert (and evangelist for separate bedrooms) says, 'sharing a bed is a cultural norm, with no science behind it. Posh people have never done it. It's a mark of wealth to sleep separately – it should be aspirational.' He says that 'sensible Victorians are said to have wailed about the intolerable cruelty of having to share a bed'.

An episode of the recent and popular Carnival Films (UK) drama *Downton Abbey*, which is set in Britain in the first two decades of the 1900s, has a scene in which the lady of the manor is in bed and her eldest daughter Mary (in her twenties and still living at home) is sitting talking to her. The Lord comes in wearing his bathrobe, prepared to come to bed. Mary asks her father, 'Dad, could you at least pretend you sleep in separate beds like normal people?' He replies, 'I keep a bed made up in my suite for the sake of propriety and that's the most you should expect.'

The ongoing evolution of the home has seen dwellings become more sophisticated and separated into designated areas for specific use – e.g. eating, living and sleeping. Cheaper housing materials and building methods have given families in developed Western societies and middle to upper socio-economic groups access to more space. This has provided more opportunities for people to enjoy their own room if desired. However, cultural, social and socio-economic factors still impact on both the choice and the reality of whether you get a bed and a room to yourself each night.

What is immutable and timeless across all cultures and civilisations is the reality that access to resources (property and money) always has and will determine the amount of space you have. In our homes, or wherever we look to lay our heads at night, there is more space and choice when we have more property and money. This is why an eight-bed dorm will always be the fate and domain of the budget traveller and the multi-room hotel suite the destination of the wealthy.

Alongside the physical evolution of where we can sleep, social evolution has seen the bed shifting from a place of protection and procreation to a more private and intimate space for two people in a relationship. The increases in moral and economic freedom seen since the middle of the twentieth century have certainly impacted on our night-time behaviours. Changing moral standards through the 1950s, '60s and '70s saw couples living together rather than marrying but enjoying all the benefits of a marriage, which include sleeping in a bed together.

And so we arrive at today, where couples share a bed as the 'cool thing to do'. But history also tells us that this isn't the only configuration that is acceptable, possible or more importantly, desirable. There appears to be no evidence to say that a couple in a bed each night is the deigned evolutionary track. I would suggest that all the evidence is to the contrary – it's what works for you and your cultural, social and economic conditions. In fact, I would hope that as we continue to evolve socially, an increasing freedom will allow us to choose where we sleep each night with no-one giving a social sneer at all. If we have the freedom to share a bed when we want to, why can't we choose not to, with equal freedom?

Cultural contrast

Outside contemporary Western society, many cultures ascribe a different meaning and importance to the 'who is where with whom and in what bed?' question. While there is a wealth of research into the science of sleep, there is a dearth of information when it comes to anthropological scrutiny over the behavioural aspect of sleeping. However, the following information provides some insight into the understanding that not all cultures view 'couple sleep' the same way.

African, Asian and South American cultures approach sleep pragmatically, with some still preferring group sleep over private spaces. How each individual, family, social group or 'tribe' approaches sleeping is based more on local and inherited practices rather than broader social norms.

> *As a couple, it's never really mattered where we sleep. Our kids have always slept with us or in our room – either on the bed or on the floor. In our family we have Italian, Malay and Aboriginal heritage and the practice of the family sleeping in various places around the house has just always been the way we 'do life' in our house. This is common practice that has been in my family for generations. My daughter is now doing the same with her first child. Her husband is Islander and they too have more a 'group' approach to who sleeps where.*
> **Dianne, educational professional, 52, married 30 years**

Japan has a strong culture of couples sleeping in separate rooms. Jay Dwivedi, a commentator on Japanese culture, reports that as many as 70 per cent of Japanese couples do not sleep together once they have a child. Before having a child, 25 per cent of the couples do not sleep together. Despite being at an age when their libidos are running wild, *Shukan Bunshun*, a popular Japanese magazine, reports that as many as three out of four couples in their twenties prefer a separate bedroom.

Marriages in which the couple do not live together are becoming increasingly common in modern Beijing, China. Guo Jianmei, director of the centre for women's studies at Beijing University, explains that, 'Walking marriages reflect sweeping changes in Chinese society.' This practice sees the husband in the couple 'walk' to his wife's family home if physical relations are sought, but there is no day-to-day domestic life, nor sharing of property.

A similar arrangement exists in Saudi Arabia. It is called a *misyar* marriage, and also involves the husband and wife living separately but meeting regularly for marital relations.

In comparison, a tribe in South Sudan (where polygamy operates) has a law that says husband and wife must sleep in the same bed. If couples don't sleep in the same bed it is seen as a sign of marital unhappiness and can be interpreted as not wanting to have sex. In this male-dominated tribe, a woman refusing to sleep with her husband will result in elders and family members getting involved to try and solve 'the problem'. Exceptions do exist for such reasons as nursing babies, pregnancy, menstruation or extreme sickness, but whatever the reason, the tribe always views the act of sleeping in separate beds as weakening the relationship.

> *If a wife does not sleep with her husband there is something wrong with the marriage. It is the law that says man and wife should sleep together. If the woman does not sleep with the man then the problem needs to be taken to the tribal elders and fixed. If my wife refuses to sleep in the same bed and have sex with me, I think she is trying to punish me. This can lead to divorce.*
> **Abedi, 38, school teacher in Sudan, married 3 years**

Religion and beds

While there do not appear to be many direct religious influences on the practice of sleeping in the same or separate beds, Klösch notes that men and women sleeping together did not always suit the moral concepts of the church. In the Middle Ages, historian Einhard (circa AD 830) warned that the bed was to provide shared accommodation for a man and a woman who were joined by love and should only be used for procreation.

Among Orthodox Jews, it is standard practice for married couples to have two beds because of Niddah (menstrual purity) laws. These laws forbid a married couple from touching each other for at least 12 days out of every menstrual cycle. To work around the laws couples will often have twin beds that they push together or pull apart as appropriate.

The Koran instructs Muslim couples to sleep separately when one is committing *nushuz*. This is where one partner in a couple is, in essence, rebelling against the confines of the marriage. Until the issue is addressed the Koran instructs husbands to 'avoid their wives in sleeping places ...' (Koran 4:34).

Some religions have dogmatic attitudes about a woman's place in marriage, namely that she is subservient to her husband. This attitude could prevent, or at least limit, a woman's ability to be assertive enough to take the steps to sleep separately, or put enormous social pressure on her to accept 'her lot'. It would be reasonable to assume that religions that allow one partner a level of control over the other could influence sleeping arrangements if the dominant person of the couple decided that sharing the bed was something they wanted to do. However, there does not appear to be a religion that makes sharing a bed at all times compulsory.

> *A Christian mind-set influences your view of marriage. Often people have engaged in Christian exchange of vows, so somewhere in their psyche and worldview is the belief that a woman belongs to a man. It's a possessive act to say 'this is where you will sleep' and my sense, when I hear women complaining about not sleeping, is that the women are contracted to that arrangement in such a way that makes it too hard for them to challenge or change it. I think that their contract is emotional, sexual, economic and religious, and I think it becomes too big to challenge it because it speaks of other*

things for both parties of a lack of voice, or a lack of opinion or 'who wears the pants'.

Neil, 46, HR executive, married 19 years

In good company

Even though sleeping apart can be a taboo subject, there are a number of famous people who are open about the practice and lead the way in debunking the myths.

The Queen of England and Prince Phillip are one of the most famous couples who sleep apart – they even have separate cabins on the Royal Yacht Britannia. Sixty four years of marriage would suggest that theirs is a successful union, if longevity is anything to go by. Following their marriage, they moved into Clarence House in 1949 and had adjacent, connecting rooms. The Queen's cousin, Lady Pamela Mountbatten, explained, 'You don't want to be bothered with snoring or someone flinging a leg around. When you are feeling cosy you share your room sometimes. It is lovely to be able to choose.'

And it's not just royalty that have taken themselves off to separate chambers. Pop culture websites reported that during their marriage, Katie Holmes and Tom Cruise didn't share a bedroom due to Tom's snoring. Apparently, even Kevin Jonas, at the tender age of 23 and only married in December 2009, sleeps separately from his wife, Danielle Deleasa, because of his snoring. Scott Disick and Kourtney Kardashian were outed as separate sleepers in an episode of *Kourtney and Kim Take New York*. *E! Online* reported in the show that the couple slept in separate beds. Disick explained, 'Just want to clear up the reason why we don't sleep in bed together. I'm not a good sleeper and with [son] Mason in bed I can't fall to sleep!'

American designer Diane von Furstenberg is another example of a woman in a loving relationship who likes to sleep apart from her husband. She sleeps above her shop in New York, while her husband lives at the Carlyle Hotel. This, she told *Town & Country* magazine, is because 'he respects me so much'.

Then there are the couples who take sleeping apart to the next level by sleeping in separate houses. Mia Farrow and Woody Allen maintained separate apartments across New York's Central Park for a number of years. People could argue that this distance may have had some impact on the events that unravelled their marriage — we'll never know.

A seemingly more successful couple who have two children, but live in separate houses, are Tim Burton and Helena Bonham-Carter. They get to watch telly together and spend time with their two children, but Helena doesn't have to tolerate Tim's insomnia, and he can close the door on her constant chatter. It works ideally, she agrees. 'I've got nothing but good things to say about it.'

In a paper considering if sleep was an activity worthy of sociological consideration, Brian Taylor suggests that we stop talking about 'being asleep' and start talking about 'doing sleeping'. His reason for this suggestion is that he proposes a 'discourse of dormancy' be created that truly brings sleep into the sociological domain. I feel that Taylor underestimates the vast number of conversations already taking place between couples and families across the world about how they 'do sleeping'.

The problem is that these conversations are not in the public domain – they are in the shared bedrooms of the world. Scientific research has focused mostly on how individuals sleep every night, while in bedrooms around the world social experiments in sleeping together are also being conducted every night. The discourse of 'will you stop that, I can't get to sleep' has been part of our language for a long time and isn't about to stop any time soon.

> **PAUSE FOR THOUGHT...**
>
> ☾ Are you aware of what the sleeping arrangements of your parents or grandparents, or older friends and relatives, are or were? If so, what are they?
>
> ☾ Are you aware of any sleeping arrangements by friends or relatives that challenge the norm of a couple sleeping in the same bed together? If so, what are they?
>
> ☾ Do you have any pre-conceived ideas about who should sleep with whom in certain social arrangements? Do you ever talk about these to others, or judge other people because of their choices?
>
> ☾ Do you know anyone whose sleeping arrangements are dictated by cultural or religious expectations?
>
> ☾ Do you or your partner have cultural or religious influences that impact on how you think about or manage your sleeping arrangements? If so, what are they?
>
> ☾ Do you ever talk to other people about any sleep-related issues? Is it common to do so in your social groups?

2

The science of sleep

'If you didn't know what sleep was, and you had only seen it in a science fiction movie, you would think it was weird and tell all your friends about the movie you'd seen.' – George Carlin

If you have been sharing a bed for ten weeks, ten months or ten years and wonder why you feel or look ten years older than you actually are, then lack of sleep could be the reason. Just as biomechanics is important for those who exercise, and food science needs to be understood for those who diet, the science behind sleep is an important factor to consider in the domain of bed sharing.

The physiology of sleep differs from person to person. Factors that impact on how our body manages sleep are hardwired into each individual's DNA and are not necessarily open for negotiation. As couples we all accept that we are not always going to like the same food, exercise at the same time (if at all), have the same religious beliefs or the same tastes in television shows. So why do we think that our sleep needs are going to be similar? Or do we even think about sleep when we set out to find a partner?

Who includes sleeping behaviours in the list of 'must haves' when considering a dream partner? I know it was never on my list. Not once did I think, 'He needs to be at least six-feet tall, handsome, dark hair, love the outdoors and need at least seven hours of sleep each night, going to bed somewhere between 9 and 10 pm.' Similarly, I doubt if 'so tell me about your circadian rhythms and melatonin production cycle' has been a popular conversation starter at speed dating events or at bars and nightclubs.

A problem with shared sleeping in blossoming relationships is that in the early days, it is often an activity of low importance. The chemicals of attraction that see us pursuing another will send couples into a blissful daze, with the practicalities of daily life ignored in favour of the more interesting activities of a new relationship. However, every relationship eventually moves into the everyday. And it is in the routine and potential monotony of life that every relationship begins to face its challenges. Once a couple starts heading to bed most nights just to sleep – rather than tear each other's clothes off with unbridled passion – is when the harsh necessities of this nightly human activity reveal their true impact.

While this book focuses on helping couples maintain their relationships despite different sleep needs, the bitter reality is that without enough sleep, we can all begin to fall apart as a person. We all need enough rest every day to give us the mental, emotional and physical strength to manage our lives. And if you are in a situation when you aren't having this each night – whatever the reason—then you might find yourself 'falling apart' both on a personal level and a relationship level.

My lack of sleep, and the effect it had on me physically, emotionally and mentally, led to me to thinking about the activity of sleep – a bit obsessively at times, I admit. When I was not getting enough sleep, I turned to research to help me understand why I felt so physically awful and mentally inept. After reading about sleep deprivation, I remember feeling a strong sense of relief that the symptoms I was experiencing, such as irritability, low energy and lack of concentration, were neither uncommon nor inconsequential.

So why all this fuss about sleep?

Without any question or doubt, human beings need sleep. Why we need sleep is a question that has challenged scientists for centuries. The earliest documented sleep theory is attributed to the Greek philosopher and physician Alcmaeon in 500–450 BC who wrote about blood flow in the sleeping body.

The scientific community admits that no definitive explanation exists about why we need to sleep despite the time spent exploring the question. What is understood and known though, is that sleep is an anabolic, or building process, that has a range of positive effects on the human body.

Positive effects of sleep

Sleep has numerous positive affects on the body, including:
- Conserving and restoring the body's energy supplies that have been depleted through the day's activities
- Providing a time for the body to do most of its repair work; muscle tissue is rebuilt and restored
- Allowing for the secretion of growth hormone, which is important for growth in children, and also important throughout adulthood to rebuild tissues
- Restoring mental energy; we spend all day thinking and creating and using our energy stores and sleep replenishes these stores
- Providing downtime for changes in the structure and organisation of the brain, a phenomenon known as brain plasticity
- Inducing the production of collagen and enhancing the skin's capacity to hold water, which are two key ingredients to

keeping your skin as close as possible to your chronological age
- Reinforcing memory and learning by allowing the brain to replay the events of the day
- Improving immune responses.

The benefits of sleep are good reason alone to get your eight hours every night. Although why we sleep is not definitively understood, there is no dispute among sleep researchers about what happens when we don't get enough sleep.

A lack of sleep has serious effects on our ability to function. Countless studies have shown that humans struggle to function if sleep deprived. In 2006 the *ICSD-II: International Classification of Sleep Disorders* distinguished more than one hundred different sleep disorders – so there's no shortage of information on what can go wrong. There are sleep foundations in most countries that research what we should and shouldn't be doing when it comes to sleep and a constant stream of findings from sleep research about the effects of too much, not enough or unusual sleeping patterns in humans.

Of particular interest to me is a recurrent finding in sleep research that when it comes to sleeping – like so many other parts of our life – men and women are different. While I am wary that this book might portray men as the villains of sleep disturbance, research findings aren't in their favour (sorry guys!). Klösch reports that while studies find only minor biological differences between men and women when it comes to how we actually sleep, a 2007 study titled 'Sex differences in the reactions to sleeping in pairs versus sleeping alone in humans' reported more discernible differences in the impact men have on women when they share a bed.

The study investigated what the actual and perceived effects of sleeping with a partner were for both men and women. John

Dittami, author of the study found, 'the bottom line is that our results indicate that women are more disturbed by the male presence in bed than the men by a woman's presence. When it came to the perceived effects, he concluded that, 'women enjoy male presence psychologically even though it costs them minutes or even hours of sleep'. There are behaviours where men are represented more prominently than women in the sport of 'waking up my partner'. These will be discussed in chapter three.

My discussions with couples over the last five years would support the findings anecdotally, but certainly not exclusively, as you will see throughout the book. We are all aware that there are many physiological differences between genders. This is just another of those areas of difference that when approached sensibly, can be noted and managed.

Issues such as sleep patterns, environmental needs and temperature issues consistently highlight an arena for the 'battle of the sexes' to continue its tournament of differences. As an example, one commonly reported gender difference is found in the contest of the light versus the heavy sleeper. Klösch[1f] explains that because of biological, cultural and social conditions, women are disposed to an increased need to control their environment, which contributes to issues with falling asleep and staying asleep as they are more sensitive to any stimuli that might wake them. In contrast, men tend to avoid or ignore stimuli and fall asleep as soon as their heads hit the pillow.

A 2012 study by the Appleton Institute at the Central Queensland University, called the 'Sealy Sleep Census Report', surveyed over 13,000 people and found that males fall asleep on average eleven minutes faster than females, and seem to be mostly untroubled after that.

Storms, pets, phones, neighbours ... nothing wakes my husband up. I would love to have his skill of putting my head on the pillow and being asleep in a nano second like he does. Honestly, I think I could take another man into bed and he wouldn't notice.
    Lulu, 42, legal professional, married 6 years

I've given up on expecting him to wake up when the kids need something during the night. I actually quite amaze myself how I can hear the slightest noise from the other end of the house. Maybe it's a superhero power I've developed. Don't think I will become famous for it though.
    Maria, 38, database analyst, married 8 years

I don't think I will revert back to where we were in the beginning with our sleeping, even when the children have grown up. I do expect that my sleeping will permanently be changed from having children and always listening out for them. I expect I will be sleeping by myself a few nights a week for ever now.
    Maree, 30, health professional, married 3 years

To further support that gender differences are indeed an issue for many couples, and backing up the 2007 survey on sex differences in sleep, a 2010 study by The American Sleep Foundation found that more than half the women they surveyed, aged eighteen to 64, said they slept well only a few nights a week because of sharing a bed. Of these, 43 per cent believed their lack of sleep interfered with their ability to deal with the next day's activities.

After two years of not sleeping properly due to my partner's snoring and movement in bed I couldn't function any more. Every day I was cranky with everyone and reached the point where I felt like I was falling apart. I started to put on weight, would go to work with an aching body, and couldn't cope with the normal pressures of life. My judgement was impaired to the point that I was so hypersensitive, I thought I was never going to sleep again.

Louise, 48, teacher, defacto for 7 years

Grumpy, irritable, indecisive, throwing tantrums ... behaviour of a two year old, right? No, this is in fact me on many given days: a 28-year-old woman that should know how to act better. But it is literally beyond my control. This is how I act when I don't get enough sleep. I have a foggy mind, I cannot concentrate, am incredibly irritable, sometimes even shaky ... it's almost like having an awful hangover every day. I remember clearly one day being so tired and getting ready for work. Suddenly I wondered what the burning sensation under my arms was only to realise that instead of deodorant I had in fact sprayed hairspray all over myself!

Emily, 30, international flight attendant, married 1 year

My husband recently talked to me about not feeling very close anymore. I was surprised by his question, but then he told me that I had been telling him to f*** off for the past week when he tried to tuck me in and cuddle me after I went to my bed. I had no idea I was doing it – I'm just so tired. I felt so bad because the cuddles when I go to my bed are really important to us.

Charlotte, 24, teacher, married 1 year

For both genders, just one night without sleep makes concentration more difficult and shortens our attention span considerably. With continued lack of sleep, the part of the brain that controls language, memory, planning and sense of time is severely affected, practically shutting down. In fact, an Australian study in 1997 discovered that only seventeen hours of sustained wakefulness leads to a decrease in performance equivalent to a blood alcohol level of 0.05 per cent – two glasses of wine and the legal driving limit in many countries.

Research also shows that sleep-deprived individuals often have difficulty in responding to rapidly changing situations and in making rational judgements. In real life situations, the consequences are grave and lack of sleep is said to have been a contributing factor to such infamous disasters as the Exxon Valdez oil spill, the Chernobyl and Three Mile Island nuclear reactor meltdowns, and the Challenger shuttle explosion.

The disasters stemming from lack of sleep are not limited to large-scale catastrophes. Bob Ellis, an Australian writer, journalist, film-maker and political commentator has noted a number of political career threatening and ending decisions and actions that he claims were due to sleep deprivation caused by plane flights. He includes Australian Prime Minister Julia Gillard's 2010 gaff in Geneva when she declared that foreign policy 'was not her passion', and the Leader of the Opposition Tony Abbott declaring at the same time in Afghanistan that 'shit happens' when asked about his thoughts on soldiers dying in the course of their duties. Neither statement set them in a winning political position, but instead left a public relations disaster for their media staff to clean up.

Although most of us do not have jobs as important as head of state, I'm sure there are times when all of us can recall putting in less than stellar performances at work or even in our relationships when in a sleep-deprived state.

My wife was due to give birth and was not sleeping well. Her tossing and turning kept us both awake for about two weeks straight. At the time, I was in charge of entering data into a database used to calculate university entrance scores of the senior students at the school where I worked. It was only the request of the Head of English for a copy of the grade's scores entered for the subject that saved the students from a

catastrophe. When entering the data I had skipped a name at the top of the list and entered all remaining scores incorrectly. In my tired state, I hadn't even picked up that I was 'out of sync' when I got to the end of the list. My mistake would have significantly impacted many students' lives and I hadn't even realised.
Warren, 52, deputy principal

Consequences of sleep deprivation

Sleep deprivation can lead to:

- Fatigue, lethargy and lack of motivation
- Moodiness and irritability
- Reduced creativity and problem-solving skills
- Inability to cope with stress
- High blood pressure
- Weakened immune system
- Reduced ability to concentrate
- Weight gain
- Cosmetic signs of premature ageing
- Increased risk of obesity
- Impaired motor skills and increased risk of accidents
- Difficulty making decisions
- Increased risk of diabetes
- Increased risk of heart disease
- Memory loss
- Possible episodes of sleep paralysis that are usually accompanied by hallucinations
- Increased likelihood of mentally 'stalling' or fixating on one thought

- Increased chance of becoming depressed.

On the issue of weight alone, a sleep study in 1984) revealed that people who averaged six hours of sleep per night were 27 per cent more likely to be overweight than those who got seven to nine hours. And those who averaged only five hours of sleep per night were 73 per cent more likely to be overweight due to an imbalance in hormones that promote hunger – in particular for simple sugars and carbohydrates – and a slowing down in the body's metabolic rate.

> *Since my husband and I moved into separate rooms I am sleeping so much better. Because of the unbroken and better quality sleep I'm getting up three mornings a week at 5.30am and exercising for an hour. Before we moved into separate rooms, I felt drained in the mornings; now I feel so rested and have energy to exercise. I'm actually losing weight.*
>
> **Anne, 44, senior manager, married 20 years**

A 2010 study at the Woolcock Institute of Medical Research, Sydney, found that during deep sleep, metabolically active hormones, such as growth hormones, are secreted. People who don't fall into deep sleep, for example people with sleep apnoea, don't get this growth hormone secreted and this can increase the risk of obesity and diabetes.

How much sleep do you need?

As well as knowing why we need sleep and what happens when we don't, there is also the question of how much sleep each person needs. Even though there is a general acceptance that we need eight hours sleep a night (drummed in to most of us since we were young) there appears to be no magic number. Just like many other unique characteristics we inherit at birth, the amount of sleep we need to function at our best varies among those who are of similar age, gender, ethnic or cultural group.

Interestingly, some cultures view sleep as a waste of time and view those people who function with minimal sleep as diligent and strong-willed.

Klösch speaks of historical writings in China, Japan and Europe, extolling the virtues of the political and clerical elite who required only a few hours of sleep. The similarity of God, who 'neither slumbers nor sleeps' (Psalm 121:3–4), to the person who could rule and lead with minimal rest each night, made eight hours each night the domain of wimps.

There are many historical figures and celebrities who are renowned for needing minimal sleep each night and this characteristic is often viewed with awe by us less famous, ordinary folk. How can someone so intelligent, productive, clever, and inspirational get by with just a few hours sleep each night? The answer is that, like supermodels, they are simply blessed with good genes.

- Thomas Jefferson – 2 hours
- Nikola Tesla – 2 to 3 hours
- Benjamin Franklin – 2 to 4 hours
- Sir Isaac Newton – 3 to 4 hours
- Florence Nightingale – 4 hours
- Michelangelo – 4 hours
- Napoleon Bonaparte – 4 hours
- Thomas Edison – 4 hours
- Jay Leno – 4 hours
- Madonna – 4 hours
- Margaret Thatcher – 4 hours
- Martha Stewart – 4 hours
- Winston Churchill – 5 hours
- Bill Clinton – 5 to 6 hours

While these people – and no doubt countless others – are able to function on minimal amounts of sleep each night, most of us tend to need a little more. If you are a person who needs a good eight hours sleep every night and are wondering why you aren't one of these superheroes who can survive on a few paltry hours of sleep each day, stop giving yourself a hard time. Researchers at the University of California, San Francisco, discovered that some people have a gene that enables them to function on only a few hours of sleep a night. But the gene is very rare, appearing in less than 3 per cent of the population; for the other 97 per cent of us, it's six hours plus each night. So put the Lycra suit away and keep your underpants on the inside.

And if you are still feeling like an underperformer because you need more than four hours a night, take heart in knowing that Albert Einstein is reported to have needed ten hours sleep each night to be well-rested and ready to solve those tricky scientific problems.

Common consensus from sleep researchers is that most healthy adults need between seven to nine hours of sleep each day. A different suggestion by Neil Stanley from the University of Surrey's sleep research laboratory puts the range at between three to eleven hours, depending on individual needs. And another view is offered by historian Roger Ekirch of Virginia Tech and psychiatrist Thomas Wehr, who both contend that a natural pattern for humans is two 'chunks' of sleep each night, punctuated by a period of wakefulness, called segmented sleeping. This may resonate with those of you who wake in the early hours of the morning, read or watch television, then fall back to sleep for three to four hours.

Age also affects the amount of sleep we require. As newborns we need up to eighteen hours sleep per day. This reduces as we age. The Division of Sleep Medicine at Harvard Medical School reports that as we get older (into our sixties, seventies and eighties) the depth of our sleep is reduced. It is common to find that any noise in the sleep environment is more likely to wake older people because of the inability to be in deep sleep as much as those who are younger.

The National Institute of Health in America points out that the best way to figure out if you're meeting your sleep needs is to evaluate how you feel as you go about your day. If you're getting enough sleep, you'll feel energetic and alert all day long, from the moment you wake up until your regular bedtime. Sounds pretty logical doesn't it?

If all that isn't enough to consider on the issue of sleep already, we have to factor in our own very unique body clock.

Each of us has an internal 24-hour sleep wake cycle, otherwise known as our biological clock or circadian rhythm. This cycle is regulated by processes in the brain that respond to how long we have been awake as well as the changes between light and dark. Some of us like to - or need to - go to bed early and wake up early; these people are often referred to as larks. Then there are those of us, the owls, who stay up late and enjoy a long lie in to ensure we get the right amount of sleep to function. Larks and owls just weren't mean to perch on the same sleeping branch.

What determines our lark or owl behaviour is the same system that regulates the cycles of many bodily functions. Our internal biological clock resides in the brain and regulates the timing of functions such as appetite, hormone release, and metabolism, as well as our sleep cycle.

An important aspect of the sleep cycle is the production of melatonin, a hormone that makes you feel sleepy. When the sun goes down and it becomes dark, the pineal gland is 'turned on' and begins to actively produce melatonin. Usually, this occurs around 9-10 pm and the increasing melatonin levels in the blood result in our beginning to feel less alert. However, the process differs from person to person, thereby causing us to feel sleepy at different times.

After we feel sleepy and head off to bed, we all fall into repetitive sleep cycles. There are five stages to the sleep cycle, each cycle lasting approximately 90 minutes. Four stages are non-REM (rapid eye movement) and one stage is REM sleep, when we do most of our active dreaming and our eyes tend to move – hence the name.

Getting good sleep is not just a matter of spending enough hours in bed. The amount of time you spend in each of the stages of sleep matters. A normal adult spends approximately 50 per cent of total sleep time in light sleep, 20 per cent in REM sleep, and 30 per cent in the remaining stages, including deep sleep – also called slow wave sleep.

Each stage of sleep in the sleep cycle offers benefits to the sleeper. However, deep sleep and REM sleep are particularly important. Those of you who have a night of broken or interrupted sleep may wake up feeling as if you haven't slept at all – even if you have been asleep for hours. If you do not reach all the stages of sleep your body may not receive all the restorative benefits of sleep required to refresh and regenerate the body. This is a really important aspect of sleep that can be problematic if you have a couple sharing a bed. One or both of you may be waking the other intermittently during the night and disturbing the other's deep sleep cycles.

Research suggests that four to five sleep cycles are needed each night for a good night's sleep – hence the recommendation of about eight hours sleep each day (seven and a half hours to be precise). Or, if you subscribe to the segmented sleeping theory, then you need two, four-hour cycles.

That's so me!

So does any of this information about sleeping touch a chord with you? Have you experienced sleep-deprivation symptoms such as forgetfulness and then worried that early dementia might be on the cards? Or do you now realise why your partner becomes upset when you happily read late into the night to their dismay and annoyance, and then find you are handed a hasty rebuke in the morning when you can't wake up to get the kids ready or head out for a 6.30 am breakfast with friends?

While it's easy to accept that your soul mate doesn't share your love of pickled herrings or competitive Frisbee, it may not be as easy to accept that this soul mate doesn't share your sleep habits and, worse still, wants to sleep apart from you as a result of your sleep habits. It's a difference many people don't like to think about, let alone talk about, but it's a reality of life that requires management.

A 2011 study supported by the National Institute of Health through the National Heart, Lung, and Blood Institute highlighted the importance of considering the interpersonal consequences of sleep and sleep loss. The study found that, among other results, the quality of interactions among married couples is affected by wives' inability to fall asleep at night but not by husbands' sleep problems. A 2009 study by the American Academy of Sleep Medicine found similar results that indicated that on a day-to-day basis, couples' relationship quality affects their sleep, and their sleep also affects their subsequent relationship functioning.

In 2012 The *Weekend Australian* newspaper reported the findings of a 1991 study by Jeffry Larson, a marriage and family therapist at Brigham Young University in Provo, Utah. The study of 150 couples found that those couples with mismatched body clocks argued more – 2.13 times per week, compared with 1.6 times per week – and spent less time together in shared activities. They also had less sex too. Larson's recommendations were that couples with differences in their sleep cycles need to accept that body clocks are hardwired and most people can't re-jig their natural bedtime and waking-up time by more than one hour.

There are many researched and documented differences between the sexes that impact on sleep needs and behaviour. But as each of us is an individual, gender is not the only cause of sleep disturbance. Same-sex couples experience similar incidences of interrupted sleep due to a partner who has different sleep patterns and idiosyncrasies. The main point to understand is that as humans, we simply don't all have the same needs for sleep. We know men and women are different in so, so many ways, sleeping is just another area that highlights the physiological differences. Klösch looks at the issue of how gender affects sleep in far more detail in *Sleeping Better Together* if you are interested in reading more about the topic.

In the end, the message from most sleep experts is that you have to accept your hardwiring when it comes to sleep and find the best ways to get the sleep you need to remain healthy. Going to bed two hours later than you would really like to, just so you can retire with your partner, is not doing either of you any favours. In fact, the chances are it will have a negative impact on your relationship in the long run.

The final demand to consider on sleep is work in contemporary society. Have you ever wished you could ask your boss if you could start work an hour or two later? I know I have. Left to wake naturally, I'm up between 7.30 and 8 am. But the reality of my life is that I need to be on a bus by 7.30 am to go to work, so it's an alarm clock every morning for me. This is a common challenge. Western work culture requires most of us to be at work between 8 and 9 am every day. The construct of the nine to five work day – so eloquently expressed by Dolly Parton – lengthened by increasing travel times created by urban sprawl, sees many people being torn from REM sleep each morning to meet their work requirements. However, for some industries, giving employees the option of arriving at a time that matches their circadian rhythms may not be practically or economically viable.

Then there are shift workers; fly-in fly-out workers; workers in industries that provide night-time services; doctors and nurses in hospitals across the world; and all the other workers such as those who keep the airline industries functioning, and have even more irregular and unconventional sleeping timeframes to deal with. Our economic evolution makes all sorts of demands upon us physically, including the need to manage our sleep well enough to work effectively throughout a long day or night. The globalisation of many companies adds an extra dimension to some workers' lives who have to factor in monitoring and interacting with markets in different time zones and catching up with co-workers who have completely opposite work/sleep lifestyles. This is one of the drivers of an increasingly common complaint about computers and smart phones becoming a 'third person' in beds across the world – an issue I discuss in the next chapter.

Tech support?

For those who have smart phones and are interested in finding out about their own sleep cycles, apps are available that monitor your sleep patterns. The information is interesting in itself, but for those who find they feel groggy on waking and are far more tired than they believe they deserve to be, apps such as 'Sleep Cycle' can tell you where you were in your sleep cycle when you woke. The app will also give you a record of how many times and how long you spent in all the sleep cycles throughout the night. I highly recommend investing in the technology.

So now that we know why we need to sleep, it's time to consider the fraught practice of bed sharing.

> **PAUSE FOR THOUGHT...**
>
> ☾ How much sleep do you need to function properly? Is this different to your partner?
>
> ☾ What are your optimal sleeping times?
>
> ☾ Are you a lark or an owl? And what is your partner?
>
> ☾ Do you prefer one long sleep, or do you wake for a noticeable period during the night?
>
> ☾ Have you ever displayed any symptoms of sleep deprivation? Are you displaying them now?
>
> ☾ Have you ever thought about and noted the different sleeping patterns or needs of your partner?
>
> ☾ If there are differences, have you named them or discussed them with your partner?

3

The truth about bed sharing

'Laugh and the world laughs with you, snore and you sleep alone.'
– Anthony Burgess

A bed has many uses. It's a place to read, throw your clothes, watch television, chat on the phone, kiss and cuddle, have sex, jump up and down, cry and feel sad. However creatively we may choose to use a bed though, there's no denying that its main use is for sleeping. And as discussed in the last chapter, the somewhat prosaic activity of sleeping is an essential daily, human activity. So, inevitably we all retire to the bedroom to get our rest.

If you are part of a couple, heading to the bedroom each night to sleep may, or may not, fill you with a sense of calm and restfulness. Not to labour a point, but falling in love with a person does not guarantee a full complement of items on the compatibility tick list. The laws of attraction that send us into the arms of another to mate don't consider a raft of incompatibilities that can bite us after the heady glow of early lust wears off.

The 2012 study by the Central Queensland University mentioned earlier found a partner in your bed is more disruptive to sleep than any other noise. In the study, 57.6 per cent respondents indicated that they slept with a partner, and, of these, 34.5 per cent indicated that their partner disturbed them while getting into bed. Forty four per cent stated that their partner disturbed them by tossing and turning, and 58.5 per cent said that their partner's snoring disturbed their sleep. Over 48 per cent said their partner disturbed them by getting up to go to the bathroom at night; 10.1 per cent reported that their sleep was disturbed by their partner getting up to go to the kitchen; 8.1 per cent of respondents were disturbed by their partner answering phone calls; and 35.9 per cent had been disturbed by a partner getting up to go to work.

Yet despite all the potential and known problems that go hand-in-hand with the activity, we keep slipping between the sheets with each other with an infallible optimism.

There are good and bad aspects to bed sharing. The critical determinant is the needs and wants of each individual and how determined that individual is to have those needs and wants met. Bedtime behaviours are in themselves mundane. But add in the human elements of temperament, emotion, power plays, relationship dynamics, traditions, morals, pride, changing attitudes, physical health and personality and a set of mundane behaviours can go from being banal to a battlefield.

As discussed, there is the expectation of couples (especially in most Western cultures) who marry or choose to live together that part of the deal of sharing your life with each other includes sharing a bed.

> *You are a married couple, you are a partnership and sleeping together is a symbol of that.*
> **Amelia, 41, mother of two, married 12 years**

> *It's a social thing that you sleep together; you're in the same room. Loving parents sleep in the same room – not separate rooms.*
> **Anne, 44, senior manager, married 20 years**

Think when you find your soulmate you go with the flow – come on you are married share a bed – not difficult. (sic)
Anonymous, www.mamamia.com.au

Being married for the first time at 44 meant it took me a while to adjust to sleeping with someone after a long time of being single and having the whole bed to myself. Despite this, I never considered not sharing a bed – for me, being married meant that as a couple we would share a bed together.
Sarah, 52, education officer, married 8 years

When my friends came out from the States in the 1990s and built a house with separate rooms, I thought their marriage was over. Word got around our friendship group and everyone talked about it and thought the same thing.
Von, 72, married 55 years

My emotional side argues that 'It's not normal if you don't sleep next to your husband. You have to make it work' and my logical side screams 'Are you crazy? You need proper sleep! If that means sleeping separately then so be it!'
Emily, 30, international flight attendant, married 1 year

I think there's something wrong. Her parents aren't sleeping in the same bed anymore.
Gretchen Wieners, Mean Girls

The good stuff

I don't deny that sharing a bed with another person provides a distinct level of intimacy to a relationship that's hard to replicate. The rituals associated with sharing a space each night, getting ready for bed, spending time alone in the sanctity of a bedroom and lying next to someone – whether you snuggle or barely touch – are part of a relationship that some couples simply could not live without.

> *I find shared sleep deeply sexy; often more so than making love. It's where true love lies, beyond words, beyond sex.*
> **Nikki Gemmel,** *The Weekend Australian Magazine,* 21-22 January 2012

> *Sharing a bed with my wife Sarah gives me a sense of completeness, togetherness and closeness. As we drift off to sleep together each night, I am reassured that all is well with the world.*
> **Thomas, 63, organisational consultant, married 8 years**

Physical contact with another human can be calming and comforting in itself and is often sought through sharing a bed and the rhythm of sleep. Many couples speak of the intimacy that bed sharing brings. This daily act can often be both a personal and public symbol of the closeness a couple shares – often because sleeping together signifies a closer liaison.

> *I enjoy the intimacy of sleeping with my partner. I sometimes like to cuddle up to her and she is receptive although she may be asleep. This behaviour is reciprocal. Sometimes we hold hands, sometimes just rest a hand on each other.*
> **Chris, 51, builder, with partner for 3 years**

> *I love ending the day next to my husband. No matter what's happened in the day ... our bed is our haven when there's just the two of us. We can share the day, plan the next day, console and cajole. We can be tender and touch or fall asleep from exhaustion with very little said but with the knowledge that we share the bed, an arm's length away and tomorrow another day.*
> **Alana, 60, personal assistant, married 32 years**

There is a social aspect to bed sharing that many couples enjoy and choose to prioritise over disrupted sleep. In fact, some may view sleeping with another person – be it a partner, child or friend – as a social event in itself. I know that there are many people who simply like sharing a bed with their partner. The cuddling and chatting, and camaraderie of hopping into this small comfy space each night has a romantic allure and can be wonderful to share with another.

Retiring to bed each night can provide the opportunity to spend quiet time together to debrief on the day, discuss topics you may not want to bring up in front of children, have a serious conversation with your partner on a personal issue, or lie quietly next to each other in that comfortable silence couples develop over time and a life shared together. In an increasingly busy lifestyle, this may be the only time when couples find the time to be alone with the other to meet a myriad of needs.

> *My wife and I are so busy in our lives, that sleeping together is often the only place we can spend time alone together. Just knowing that I can at least touch her hand and lie next to her is all I need to reconnect each day. I couldn't live without it.*
>
> **Tony, 47, IT consultancy business development manager, married 25 years**

> *I cherish my time in bed with my partner. I love our little chats before we fall asleep. I love his snuggles in the middle of the night. To the point where I can't sleep if he's not in bed with me.*
>
> **Trina, www.mamamia.com.au**

> *The one thing I look forward to at the end of each day is the brief moment, before we go to sleep, when I get to lay my head on my husband's chest and hear his heart beating. We don't talk. But just that brief connection means so much to me. Sleeping together gives us the chance for regular intimacy such as midnight discussions about topics that worry us. Sometimes you can talk about things so much easier when lying next to one another in the dark. Quite often we will hold hands while we are talking about things that worry us and this is reassuring.*
>
> **Cass, www.villainouscompany.com**

Sleeping with another person may also be an activity that is habitual. Individuals who slept with siblings in a bed or a room as they were growing up may equate safety and security with having another person in close proximity during sleep. There is a gender ideology that women need the protection of men, and this protection may extend to bed sharing.

> I actually sleep *better* with my partner in the bed. I don't think he makes a physical difference, but there's something comforting about him being there. I find it really hard to sleep by myself now, if I'm staying at my parents' or overnight at a party. I almost never wake up refreshed if I've slept alone.
> Shannon, www.mamamia.com.au

> I always go to bed well before my partner so I fall asleep fine by myself, but if he's away and I know he's not coming to bed that night, I can't get to sleep at all! I have to have the tv on in the other room, I hate sleeping when there's no-one else in the house.
> Alena, www.mamamia.com.au

Paul Rosenblatt, author of *Two in Bed: the Social System of Couple Bed Sharing*, says that the cited benefits of sleeping with another are either person-focused, such as warmth, sense of safety and companionship, or couple-focused, such as intimacy, shared experiences and reaffirming the couple's commitment. For those individuals who need a sense of safety security and companionship, sharing a bed can provide this and create an environment conducive to a good night's rest.

So while there is much that is good, even great, about sleeping with another, there are aspects of the practice that leave a lot to be desired. As sleeping is such a fundamental human need, honestly examining the unpleasant realities of sleep is as important as enjoying the upside.

The bad stuff

Being in close physical contact with any person, in any setting, for an extended period of time inevitably creates issues. Lying next to the same person night after night can be a breeding ground for all that can be unpleasant between two people. And while there are behaviours and habits our partners have that we can learn to live with, such as leaving the lid off the sauce bottle, or not making the bed first thing in the morning, a 1999 study by the Mayo Clinic found that people don't automatically adjust to sleep disturbances.

Even though Paul Rosenblatt[2] encourages couples to learn to sleep together, he notes the following about sharing a bed: 'Sleeping together is an achievement of coordination on many dimensions – where to locate one's head, body, arms and legs, where to put one's pillow, how to relate to the blankets, when to talk and not talk, when to touch the other and when not, how to touch the other, what ways of expressing displeasure with the other are acceptable and work, how free one is to toss and turn, what to do when the other makes noise, what to do and not do if one awakens during the night.'

It all sounds like such hard work, doesn't it?

And while each couple faces its own particular proximity issues, there do appear to be some clear winners in the litany of complaints from bed sharers. I'm going to look at the 'bad' parts of bed sharing in two categories. First, there are the actual *in-bed* bed behaviours, and then there are the habits and behaviours *around* going to bed.

Snoring

Snoring is by far the most common reason why one partner will disturb the other's sleep. And, sorry guys, but it does tend to be men who are most guilty on this charge. The National

Sleep Foundation of America supports this stain on your good characters.

> *Persons most at risk are males and those who are overweight, but snoring is a problem of both genders, although it is possible that women do not present with this complaint as frequently as men.*

The physical and medical reasons for snoring are complex and varied. They range from having one too many alcoholic drinks to life-threatening conditions such as sleep apnoea. So whether it's the man or the woman snoring in bed, it's a very common problem and it keeps a lot of people awake. Snoring also becomes more prevalent and louder as we age. And that's for both men and women. So if you are smugly reading this and have not yet reached your forties – it's all ahead of you.

> *I hated my husband because of his snoring. I hated that he could keep me awake and not even know he was doing it. When I would kick him and say 'Please stop snoring' he would say, 'I'm not snoring – what are you talking about?' and then it would be my problem and I would be furious with him. We could not have stayed in the same bed together because I really resented him for it. I resented the way he reacted. He didn't wake up and say 'I'm really sorry keeping you awake' he would wake up and say 'Stop kicking me – why are you kicking me?' and then resent me.*
>
> **Frances, 40, mother of 3, married 10 years**

> *When my husband snores I want to say 'go away you sound like a troll'. I think snoring is one of the most unattractive things a person can do. To me, it's a hideous sound and there's nothing appealing about someone who snores. So if I can't hear his snoring he looks much nicer and much more appealing to me.*
>
> **Rebecca, 47, counsellor, married 20 years**

My snoring simply became an issue for us. John tried ear plugs, but he couldn't wear them for more than three nights in a row and I felt bad that he had to.
   May, 66, retired, married 40 years

I sleep in a separate room from my partner of more than 20 years because of his snoring. We downloaded an app that measures decibels and his snoring was at the same sound level as a food processor makes grinding nuts!
   Anonymous, www.mamamia.com.au

My father's snoring eventually ended our family holidays in caravans. My brother and I would be up in the annexe at 2 am playing cards because Dad's snoring was as loud as a train.
   Kate, 46, lawyer, married 12 years

My mother is renowned for her snoring. To the point where I can only describe it as a whipper snipper next to you! And she snores no matter what, front, back and sides! My father's only saving grace is he falls asleep really quickly and easily so it's usually not a problem.
   Trina, www.mamamia.com.au

Unfortunately, snoring is something over which we have little control. While intermittent snoring can be controlled through a few less beers or wines, for many people it is embarrassing and a source of frustration. It is a pity that an unintended behaviour can have such a big impact on so many couple's lives. But I must confess that when I hear people tell of years of no sleep due to a snoring partner, I am genuinely mystified that they have done nothing to address the situation and continue to complain of no sleep.

While your partner may only emit a gentle purr that disturbs you occasionally, the voracity with which some people snore can be quite alarming. The average snorer emits a noise level of 50 decibels. This is equivalent to the noise generated by a normal conversation at home or a large electrical transformer 100 feet away. *The Guinness Book of Records* reports Koere Walkert from Sweden as one of the loudest snorers. Measured at 93 decibels on 24 May, 1993, his snoring is as loud as a belt sander. However, Walkert is a lightweight compared to Jenny Chapman in Britain, who was recorded snoring at 111.6 decibels at a snoring boot camp in 2009. This puts her as just a little louder than a chain saw, not quite as loud as a hammer drill, but still 8 decibels louder than a low-flying jet.

As a guide, anything over 70 decibels is when hearing can start to be damaged – so spare a thought for Jenny Chapman's husband. Sensibly though, he does often sleep in another room, with both bedroom doors shut and sometimes with his head under a pillow.

And fortunately for Jenny, she wasn't married to John Wesley Hardin. An outlaw who lived in America in the late 1800s, Hardin reportedly shot a sleeping stranger in the room next to him because his snoring was keeping Hardin awake. While many of us may have thought of such extreme action as well, fortunately for thousands of snorting and snuffling partners we have exercised far greater restraint.

Movement

Movement in bed can range from innocent repositioning for comfort, through to restless leg syndrome and flailing limbs that can turn the bed into a nightly replay of a good old-fashioned gladiator epic. Some people find they have partnered with a 'floundering whale' who flops around the bed all night, taking the sheets and blankets with them, oblivious to the innocent soul shivering on the other side, fuming quietly or whimpering sadly.

The reality is that sleeping involves movement, especially during the light sleep stages. We all change sleeping position around 20 times a night but Professor Jim Horne, director of Loughborough University's Sleep Research Centre, notes that men seem to shift around more than women. In an experiment conducted at the centre, movement sensors placed on men and women found that men move around twice as much in the night. This fact may help settle some arguments about the mystery of bedclothes that go awry on a nightly basis.

And while innocent and simple movement might just be annoying, sharing a bed with a 'human windmill' can be life threatening. There are documented cases of women who have bruised breasts from being rolled on during sleep. Ouch!

> *I like a lot of personal space. I like to sleep in different positions. On my back, on my tummy, arms behind my head, arms to my side, arms straight up like a soldier (rarely, but I like to keep my options open), legs splayed, knees drawn up to my chest, hanging from the chandelier wearing bunny ears and a tail (okay, so that one is my husband's fantasy). I don't like to be restricted in my movements by anyone pushing my limbs out of the way when I fancy a good stretch.*
>
> **Kerri, 44, author and blogger, with husband 20 years**

> *My husband and I regularly, accidently punch or elbow each other in the face at night. We have a queen size but I think we need to upsize to avoid injury.*
>
> **littlemisschloe, www.mamamia.com.au**

> *Where do I begin? I have been elbowed and kicked more times than I can remember, had his arm 'thud' on me as he turns over, and pushed with such force that I am jolted out of sleep with such a startle I find it hard to get back to sleep sometimes. I know he doesn't mean to do it and is always apologetic, but I*

often wonder if it would be a legal reason to justifiably let me hurt him.

Chloe, 32, accountant

Night-time comfort breaks

Another common movement during the night is one partner getting up to go to the toilet. The increase of ensuite bathrooms in modern houses mean that not only is there disruption in the act of getting out of bed, there can also be some disturbingly audible proof of the activity. For men sharing a bed with a pregnant woman, frequent toilet trips during the night – while good training for the sleeplessness to come – can be equally as disturbing.

> *While I understand that my husband needs to go to the toilet during the night, must the activity involve the broken waterfall effect, a couple of farts and that much sighing? It's always been a bone of contention between us. He won't even shut the door – 'it takes too much time'.*
>
> **Sue, 48, married 12 years**

> *I know it's wrong to be angry about things related to pregnancy, but my wife would go to the toilet about 5–6 times a night in the last couple of months of her pregnancy. I was too frightened to tell her that it was really disturbing my sleep. I just drank a lot of coffee at work. It wasn't a great time.*
>
> **Simon, 43, IT manager**

> *About 6 months into my pregnancy I just moved out into the other room. That way I could spread out, toss and turn and go to the toilet as many times as I needed.*
>
> **daisy123, www.mamamia.com.au**

Temperature

The different preferences in sleeping temperature is another way to heat things up in the bedroom, whether talking about bed coverings, breezes through an open window or air conditioning.

Research suggests that men don't perceive temperature as sensitively as women, which is why they feel warmer. One theory is that women tend to have more blood circulating around their core organs, and less around their extremities such as their hands and feet, which are the body's temperature sensors.

Hands up, those ladies who have slipped their cold feet or hands on to body parts of their male partner to warm them? I know I do it in winter (to much loud protest) when I slip in to my husband's bed for a cuddle before heading to my bed for the night. Similarly, hands up, guys who hate it when your female partner tries to suck the warmth from you with their cold hands or feet? And girls, who hasn't had a bit of a giggle when angling your cold bottom into your partner's warm embrace for a quick spoon before you slip off to sleep? Yes, it's all good fun, until one of you feels that you are being used as a human water bottle.

Typically, women prefer their sleeping environment to be warmer than men. This is backed up by Paul Rosenblatt's research; he found that 75 per cent of the heterosexual couples he interviewed reported that when one of them was warmer than the other, it was usually the man. But not always. A woman can be the partner generating the most heat. A 2001 study found that women's body temperature rises by as much as one degree towards the end of their menstrual cycle. Hormonal changes during pregnancy and menopause can also lead to a raised temperature.

> *My husband and I have had trouble sleeping together. I tend to sleep 'hot' and prefer a thinner blanket, while he sleeps 'cold' and likes a giant quilt. It took two and a half years, but we*

realised along the way that instead of a nightly debate over whose favourite blanket we would use, we would each cram our own onto the bed. We no longer have the 'your blanket makes me too hot/cold' discussion in the morning.

Kate, www.mamamia.com.au

My wife requires more warmth in the bed. She needs a doona most nights to sleep under but I want to toss it off. Each person requires their own comfort level.

Bruce, 68, married 3 years

I was undergoing chemotherapy and radiation and became impossible to sleep with. My changes in body temperature became a big issue for us both and part of the raft of reasons we moved to separate beds.

Brooke, 52, education professional, married 30 years

My husband likes to be very scientific about things. So when I reach for an extra blanket, wriggle my icy feet and complain 'it's cold ...' he'll look at the thermometer he has nearby for just such occasions and tell me that it's not cold, because it's 20 degrees in the bedroom. Different people just feel the cold differently. I can see that from my kids – one cocooned under a mound of blankets, the other spreadeagled on top of the sheets. When you are sharing a bed though, that can be tricky. I have surrendered any notion of enjoying an electric blanket. He tolerates the doona in winter, so long as most of the feathers have been distributed away from him. Little by little, we have reached an accommodation about the arrangement of blankets – and the desirability of bed socks – even though I know we will never agree on whether it is 'cold'.

Kate, 46, lawyer, married 12 years

Breathing

Whether we are asleep or awake, respiration just keeps on happening. Like snoring, this is an uncontrollable behaviour as we don't know that our mouth falls open after we fall asleep. However, as the wee hours of the morning approach, the wafting smell or the raspy sound of a loved one's breath are less than welcome.

> *After 15 years and three kids together a queen bed just doesn't cut it, when it is time to sleep I need my space! I have to face away from my hubby while sleeping, I hate being breathed on! I have actually said to my hubby that things would be a lot better if he didn't breathe overnight! Daytime breathing only!*
>
> **Sarah, www.mamamia.com.au**

> *I hate, hate, hate being breathed on! I tell Mr W he is like a dragon breathing on my neck and the sound is like a plane taking off in my ear!*
>
> **Whippersnapper, www.mamamia.com.au**

> *A king sized bed has made the sleeping experience better. In our queen sized bed I always woke up with a cricked neck from sleeping facing away from him as I hate being breathed on in the night.*
>
> **Anonymous, www.mamamia.com.au**

Like snoring, poking and prodding might make the problem of a partner breathing in your direction stop, but just like snoring, for how long? I do wonder if Darth Vader ever shared a bed with a partner?

Children and pets

Those who follow through on the laws of attractions and produce children often face additional demands on their bed real estate. Not only do you have to share with your loved one, you may have to share your minimal and prized space with some little loved ones as well.

For some, bed space may progress from a small crib, to a bigger cot, to a single bed, to a double or queen bed – all by yourself. Then you start sleeping with your partner and your bed space is halved, then the children come along and you find yourself gripping on for dear life to the last foot of space at the edge of the mattress as the toe nails of your toddler rake your calves.

The balancing act of trying to allow everyone in a family to get enough sleep often forces the hand of many parents who give in and let children share their bed.

> *After years of bed hopping to accommodate our two children who would not spend a full night in their own bed, we gave in and just started sleeping with one child in our bed and one of us in the spare bed in their room. It's been close to 10 years now and even after recently paying them $5 a night to sleep in their own bed, after about four weeks, the eldest boy started coming through to our room again, so we are back to sleeping apart.*
>
> **Michael and Liza, 41 and 39, married 10 years**

> *My partner and I have been together 8 years and slept in separate rooms for about 3 years now. I used to and probably still would love sleeping with him but since we have had kids, 2 boys within 15 months that both co-sleep, I've shifted to the spare room. We have a king-sized bed but I was still constantly annoyed and as a result, waking up shirty too. He loves the kids in the bed and it honestly doesn't bother him if he is woken up by a foot in the face or a cry for a cup of milk. I used to feel guilty but now I don't, I realise sometimes you gotta do what you gotta do!*
>
> **Lola, www.mamamia.com**

The one positive aspect of this shared-sleeping problem is that it has an end point. Most parents can be confident that they won't have to co-sleep with, or make room in their bed for, their teenager. At least, one hopes not.

There are people who could easily substitute 'pet' for 'child'. In fact, I'll bet there are some who have done it already. Some of us are more than happy to share our beds each night with a furry creature but others think that any animal in the bed is a non-negotiable 'no'.

So what happens when you meet your soulmate, and the whirlwind romance leads you to the bedroom to find that Fluffy gets to sleep in the middle of the bed, and then at the bottom, and then in the middle again, and then back to the bottom each night? Because humans can become terribly attached to their animals, this issue can be as significant as the arguments for or against children sleeping in bed.

To cuddle or not to cuddle

Is your idea of sleeping heaven when your partner takes you in their arms and holds you tight through the night until dawn's rays slip through the curtains the next morning? Or does this scenario fill with you dread, make your hands shake wildly at your side, and make you feel icky and want to say 'ewwwww'?

Just like we have different tolerance levels about activities such as holding hands and cuddling and kissing in public, some of us don't want to be held in a loving embrace all night. Because men generally fall asleep faster, women can be left trapped under a well-meaning but vice-like arm. There is also the problem of ongoing physical contact creating sweaty bodies that are neither pleasant to feel or smell, nor great for the sheets.

Spooning your loved one as you succumb to blissful slumber makes for a great visual in the movies, but doesn't really accommodate the human need for changing positions as we cycle through our sleep patterns every night.

> *I'm at the start of the trying to convince a newish boyfriend that sleeping separately is okay. Yes, I love the snuggling and the cuddling, but when it's time to sleep I really dislike being touched. I'm a light sleeper and have rheumatoid arthritis so it's hard for me to get comfortable enough to sleep well at the best of times. Having a boyfriend who feels the constant need to be touching me somehow rather complicates things. It's a really hard topic to discuss with him without feeling like I'm being cold or mean!*
>
> **Em, www.mamamia.com.au**

> *I like to cuddle up to my wife's back as we fall asleep together – I think it's called spooning. After enjoying this for about 5 minutes, I face reality, roll over, and arrange my 3 pillows the way I need them so I can sleep comfortably.*
>
> **Max, 43, company director, married 18 years**

Other in-bed sleeping problems

While I could fill a good portion of this book with what can go wrong when lying in a bed next to another, I'll leave the discussion there and leave you with a list of further complications that can be found between the sheets. The list is not definitive, which is why there are some spaces at the bottom to fill in the ones you think I've missed.

- The size of the bed
- The firmness of the bed
- Who gets to sleep on which side of the bed
- Sheet textures
- Amount and size of pillows

- Different sleep positions
- Teeth grinding
- Sweating
- Getting up in the middle of the night (not just for the toilet)
- Waking from dreams and nightmares
- Going to bed angry
- Sleep walking
- Sleep talking
- Insomnia
- Illness – temporary or long term
- _____
- _____
- _____

As well as nightly tussles when in the bed, there are also the tussles that happen before you even reach the bed or turn out the light.

As outlined in the last chapter, sleeping needs differ from person to person. If you are lucky enough to share similar sleeping needs in regards to getting ready to sleep, the time you go to bed and how long you need to sleep, then well done. However, the reality for many is that they have different bedroom behaviours that can wear down a once happily-shared activity.

Preparing to sleep

Human behaviour is swathed in habit and ritual. Learned behaviours that are replayed consciously, or that happen without much thought at all, guide us through each day, week, month and year. When it comes to going to bed, having a ritual or routine is something that begins when we are babies and don't have the slightest idea of the conditioning to which we are being exposed. Cultural factors vary, but I am sure many of you have experienced the practice of children having a set bedtime routine that involves a bath, a story reading and then being tucked into bed nice and early. This traditional approach to our early sleeping behaviour is often the origin of the rituals we adopt as we grow older, which leads me to the first, very common habit that people have when it comes to going to bed – reading before sleeping.

Similar to snoring, to read or not to read before sleep is a common battle fought out in beds across the world. The Big Sleep Survey conducted in 2010 in Australia, with over 12,000 people participating, found that 40 per cent of people like to read when they go to bed, while the Central Queensland University study reported that 59.7 per cent of people like to read in bed. Both results are significant. Reading in bed is a disruptive activity (for the sleeping party) that involves having a light on as well as movement and sound (from the page turning).

> *Having a room of one's own was a revelation. First, there was the realisation that I could read as long as I wanted, even with the main light on if I so desired. I've always read in bed – right from the days when I used to hide a flashlight under my pillow so I could continue after my mother had pronounced: 'Lights out.' But during the years of sharing a bed with David, this habit had become one of our great bones of contention: 'Can't you turn off the light? I can't sleep.' Even a specially purchased, tiny light that hooked over the cover of the book was too much for him. He would complain he couldn't sleep, and when I hid it over the edge of the bed, ruining my eyesight in the gloom, he would whine, 'But I can hear you turning the pages!' But then he liked to fall asleep with the radio on, and you can't*

concentrate on your own novel when Radio 4's 'Book at Bedtime' is burbling in the background. Now, though, I can do as I please.
  Dame Jenni Murray, British journalist and broadcaster for *The Guardian*

My husband is a shift worker, which is an issue. Being an 'owl' I never felt that I could go in to my bedroom and feel free to do anything. No activity with noise was allowed and no reading could happen because there was to be no light in the room. I missed reading in bed.
  Anne, 44, senior manager, married 20 years

Neil is a reader and I can't sleep with the light on. When he would read all night because he couldn't sleep, I would go to the spare room. Now though, he will mostly go to the spare room to read as he needs to, to help him get back to sleep.
  Ann, 46, HR professional, married 19 years

As we got older and I became more liberated, I thought why should I have to go to bed when he wants to go and why should I have to turn the lights off when he wants to go to sleep. If I wanted to continue to read he would complain about the light from my table light keeping him awake.
  Von, 72, married 55 years

Watching television in bed is another activity that some find relaxing and soporific, and others find anything but. A 2009 study of 21,475 adults by the Division of Sleep and Chronobiology at the University of Pennsylvania found that television viewing is the most dominant pre-sleep activity, accounting for almost 50 per cent of pre-bedtime, a statistic which was repeated in the Central Queensland University study. The topic even featured prominently in the movie *Sex in the City 2*: Carrie was most unhappy when Big decided to install a television in the bedroom of their New York apartment.

Television creates light and sound and causes similar problems to reading between couples.

> *I will never cease to be amazed at how my wife's interest in crappy TV increases in direct proportion to how late at night it is. She will be fighting to stay awake, but intent on getting to the end of another 'Celebrity Something' show no matter what the cost is next morning. The hum of the TV keeps me awake in itself, even without any volume. I will sometimes fall asleep on the couch just to avoid watching the rubbish. It really annoys me but she insists it helps her sleep. I think it just helps her stay awake.*
> **Wilson, 43, married 15 years**

> *TV had a great bearing on us moving to separate rooms. Margaret had a TV in the bedroom and I hated it. Absolutely detested it. Why? When I go to bed I go to bed to sleep. If I want to watch TV I can do it in the lounge room. When I wanted to go to sleep Margaret would have to turn the TV off and go out to the lounge room to continue watching her show. And then she would disturb me when she came back to bed.*
> **John, 58, building contractor, married 30 years**

> *My husband watches TV to wind down and fall asleep. The problem was that he would lie on the couch to watch TV, fall asleep, but when he woke up, turned the TV off and walked down the hall to come to bed, he would be too awake to fall asleep again. He just stays on the couch now.*
> **Suzette, 40, administrative assistant, married 17 years**

Then there are those who can't face eight hours of slumber without nourishment and take a snack to eat and/or drink when they hop in to bed. Despite the risk of crumbs or drips and drops of food in the bed and on the bedclothes, an American study found 32 per cent of people polled take meals and snacks to bed.

> My husband eats in bed, which I cannot stand. He leaves plates and bowls and water bottles by the bed. I love lovely linen and every time I bought new linen it would have chocolate ice cream or chocolate on it, which would never come out. I don't have that now, because he is eating in his bed, in his room.
>
> **Anne, 44, senior manager, married 20 years**

Staying connected

Developments in contemporary living create new challenges for the modern couple; an array of devices such as iPads, laptops, notebooks, iPhones, Galaxies, and Kindles are now a feature of pre-sleep activity. For some couples, it's not just pre-sleep either, but also during the night and first thing in the morning. Wireless networks are commonplace in homes and have given technology addicts the ability to be online anywhere and anytime.

Almost a third of participants in the 2010 Australian Big Sleep Survey keep a mobile phone in the bedroom at night, with TVs, laptops, iPods and radios found in roughly 15 per cent of bedrooms. In 2011, Ikea conducted a study of two million people and found that 22 per cent admitted to using a computer in bed (the Central Queensland University study reported 77.9 per cent of respondents said they used a computer in bed).

Compelling and arguably important reasons such as checking emails, Facebook and Twitter updates, financial information and sport results are the most common reasons for justifying the need to take a device to bed. And it's not just the fact that your partner is more interested in the screen than you, it's the audible detritus that comes with the electronica.

> *My husband has headphones listening to music when I am trying to sleep. I can still hear the music and it drives me nuts.*

> *(I think it is very anti-social for him to have headphones in bed!)*
>
> **Anonymous, www.mamamia.com.au**

> *The iPad is the third person in our relationship. Morning, noon and night my partner is emailing friends, work colleagues and all the other stuff like Facebook and the web. He knows I don't like the iPad being used in bed, but thankfully I mostly fall asleep and it doesn't disturb me.*
>
> **Pete, 32, banking professional**

Just as books create noise when pages are turned, devices will bing and beep with alerts; click when keyboards are used, and throw out a luminous glow that can light up a room just as much as a bedside light. I enjoy being able to sit in bed and use my laptop when needed, and I often watch videos on my iPhone. My husband is very attached to his iPad and seeing him lying in bed using it last thing at night and first thing in the morning is not uncommon.

If this is the area that troubles you most, there is a comprehensive study available that was done by the Sleep Foundation in America in 2011 about devices in the bedroom.

Light and sound

A dark, quiet room is the Gold Standard for sleeping. How quiet is quiet though? And how dark is dark? The earlier chapter on the science of sleep touched on the answer for why we prefer a dark environment, but it's a little bit of a 'chicken and egg' question. As melatonin is produced in the body when it gets dark, this means that we tend to sleep when it's dark; and we also need darkness to produce the melatonin to make us sleepy. Prior to the invention of electricity, artificial light didn't confuse our melatonin production so more people retired to bed earlier. Also, without electricity there weren't as many nighttime activities anyway, so going to bed was the preferred option for most people.

A recent US study found that sleeping in a room with too much light can cause depression. Scientists that conducted the study found that 'even just the glow from leaving the television on while you sleep can be enough to trigger the effect and a lack of darkness during sleeping hours can cause changes to the brain and depressive symptoms'. There are people who do not like a totally dark room, possibly the result of having a night light as a child, and equally, there are those who cannot bear even a sliver of light disturbing their sleep.

Noise in the bedroom can take many forms. I have already touched on issues such as noise from the turning of a page and noise from electronic devices. However, on the opposite end of the spectrum, there are people who like to have constant noise while they sleep. A commonly sought noise is the constant hum of an air conditioner or a fan. For some, this is more than just a temperature issue, it's that they can't sleep without some type of noise in the bedroom – they cannot 'do' quiet. Our individuality dictates the degrees of dark and quiet we need to create our optimal sleeping environment.

> *While not my story, I clearly remember a school friend's sister who slept with clocks in her room. We're not talking a couple: if memory serves, it was over 20. All clocks were ticking clocks and I was always fascinated by how she could possibly sleep at night. Being a light sleeper, it has been a story that has stayed with me. As she was unmarried at the time I knew her, I used to think about what her husband would say and do when she eventually married. I still do.*
>
> **Holly, 33, British public servant**
>
> *I cannot sleep without the fan on in the room. It's not only the feeling of the air moving over my body, but the constant hum*

that it makes. For me, that 'hum' drowns out any other noise that might keep me awake.
   Brian, 47, transport worker, married 22 years

Up and go

How do you like to be woken in the morning? By a pair of twittering bluebirds gently rousing you from your night of slumber with their songs? Or by the shattering blast of a hard rock radio station so that you know for sure you are going to stay awake? Are you a serial snoozer who has to hit that button for another 10 minutes of sleep so many times that you struggle to make the bus each day? Or are you a lark who went to bed so early that dawn's first light woke you and allowed you to pop out for a quick half hour run before most of us even realised it was day?

How we are woken can impact on our mood and attitude right from the second we open our eyes. As noted, being woken at the wrong time in your sleep cycle can leave you feeling out of sorts and struggling to get your eyes open and find your nice inner person. If you've ever been accused of 'getting out of bed on the wrong side', it could be attributed to when you were woken rather than where you were in the bed.

If a couple retire to bed at different times, but wake at the same time, the nature of sleep cycles adds an additional level of complexity to sleeping together. If one of the couple is in the middle of a deep sleep cycle when awakened, they may find it difficult to adjust immediately and feel groggy and disoriented for several minutes. This disorientation could be the reason why you're getting out of bed on the wrong side!

When my alarm goes off in the morning sometimes, it takes me forever to get my act together. I call it 'cotton wool brain', but it can sometimes last all morning. A couple of times that I have

> been up early to take people to the airport, I have had to go back home and sleep more because I know I haven't actually woken up yet. I can drive and talk and do all that, but I'm not 100%.
> **Lulu, 42, legal professional, married 6 years**

Similarly, being woken by a loud, unpleasant sound might just really annoy you, irrespective of which sleep cycle you are in.

My ex-boyfriend Brent wanted the radio alarm clock tuned to a hard rock radio station. I hated it. We agreed to swap every fortnight to the radio station of my choice, but on the mornings when a song I disliked (of which there were many) blasted me awake, it immediately put me in a bad mood. Similarly, the roles were reversed when my station was the wake-up call. Could we have chosen another way to wake up? Possibly, but two strong personalities don't always search for a rational solution. And my ongoing sleep deprivation from having to share a bed with him did not make me the most rational person at the time.

As with the 'in-bed' behaviours, I'm sure there are more personal quirks and proclivities that manifest themselves in the bedroom and serve to disturb a sleeping or attempting to sleep partner. However, I'm going to move on to the behaviours that some folk don't really like to talk about in nice company, but we all know happen when the sun goes down and we head to our bedrooms.

The stuff we don't really like to talk about

There are some human bodily functions and activities that we all know about, but don't like to mention. A few of these activities take place in the bedroom, and in the bed, and it's time to talk frankly about them.

Beeping your own horn

Animals do it. Humans do it. Apparently, humans do it on average 14 times a day. It's a natural bodily process of which we shouldn't be ashamed. It makes some people laugh uproariously and embarrasses others. It can be innocent and private or offensive and very public. Yep, I'm talking about passing wind, or, to be very blunt, farting.

On the list of bodily functions we can't control, this one sits on the margins. While the passing of wind can happen unknowingly during sleep, I know of many people who boast of producing redolent emissions in the bed and the effect it has had on a poor, unsuspecting partner. I have endured such behaviour and fail to see the humour in the act, but that's just me. This does tend to be a behaviour that amuses and entertains men more than women – if you question my gender bias on this claim, just search 'farting in bed' on YouTube.

Unfortunately for men, physiologically they are more prone to farting because they generate more gaseous product in a day than women, and this gas is released when they are most relaxed. This, even more unfortunately for their partners, is likely to be in bed.

While farting when both parties are awake is bad enough, farting while asleep constitutes cruel and unusual punishment.

> *Among a raft of behaviours that made me decide that I needed to sleep separately from my husband, his farting used to really, really irritate me. I should not have to put up with the smell of his fetid bowels when I am trying to go to sleep. As crude as that might be, it made me angry when he did fart in bed and even angrier when he thought it was funny. Even after six years of having separate bedrooms, he still thinks it amusing to come in*

to my bedroom at night, pass wind, and then leave me with the smell. There aren't words to capture how furious I become.
    Holly, 33, British public servant

When sleeping with my husband, there is always the chance I will be woken by what I call a 'vivid' dream. I'm in a deep slumber and having an amazing dream and thinking 'Wow this dream is so real! I can even smell everything' only to be slowly drawn out of my slumber to find that the 'vivid' smell in my dream is in fact real and is coming from my perfectly undisturbed peacefully sleeping husband lying next to me!

    So after letting out a frustrating 'argh!' and purposefully waking up my husband giving him a good shove, because why should he have the luxury of sleeping while I have to deal with his smell, I grab my pillow in a fit of anger and traipse off to the spare room to try to salvage a few hours of solid sleep before my alarm is due to go off.
    Emily, 30, international flight attendant, married 1 year

You know what? I sleep so much better when a man is not in my bed. My husband used to fart constantly, and it was really upsetting to me – smelly, gross and he stopped apologising too, so it was bad manners.
    Anonymous, www.mamamia.com.au

It's one of life's little luxuries.
    Ian, 42, electrician, married 5 years

The wet spot

When the activity and passion of sex is over and a couple is basking in the afterglow of their encounter, there can be an issue that takes the shine off both love and lust – the wet spot.

For some couples, who sleeps in the wet spot is not an issue at all. The post-coital bliss may be so overpowering that falling asleep with each other comes naturally and without a second thought to the state of the sheets. But for others, it can make for an uncomfortable night's sleep – especially on cold winter nights.

The wet spot can vary in size, depending on the enthusiasm of the sexual act and if a condom was used. So if there is a moist area on the sheets, after each partner's breath has returned to normal and all the brain chemicals and feel-good after effects of sex start to kick in and sleep is washing over both of you, there is the inevitable battle of who gets to sleep in the dry part of the bed – or more importantly, who doesn't.

For those among us who are practical beings, preventative measures can be taken to mitigate the effects of the wet spot. Strategically placing a towel can help with absorption, but it's not very romantic and may take away from the spontaneity of the event. Having a spare sheet ready to quickly pop on the bed can also help, but again it's not really what most of us want to be doing after we've had sex.

Women may think that the chivalrous thing to do is for the man to valiantly offer up the dry area for his partner, but in these days of equality, that approach may be seen as untrue to the philosophies of the women's liberation movement.

Nine times out of ten, I will end up lying in the wet spot after sex. My partner falls asleep so quickly after sex, and it's a deep sleep that I can barely wake him from. I don't think he does it on purpose, but there have been many times that I have found a towel or a nighty to put over the spot so it's not so 'icky'. I know it sounds a bit whingy, but after six years together the romance is waning a bit and it's hard to not get practical about these things.

Sam, 32, administrative assistant

> *My wife makes a bit of a deal about the wet spot sometimes and will make me swap sides of the bed so that I have to sleep in it. I fall asleep quickly anyway, but I don't like not sleeping on my side of the bed.*
> **Ben, 36, builder**

Sleeping separately will not completely stop the issue of the wet spot either – it just splits it across two beds. The problem that separately sleeping couples may face is whose bed is going to be subjected to the possibility of the wet spot.

> *There have been a couple of times after I have put clean sheets on my bed that I have manoeuvred to have sex with my husband in his bed rather than mine. It took him a while to work it out, and then he started doing it too. 'Whose bed will have the spot' doesn't stop us having sex, but it makes choosing the location a bit more strategic. We mostly laugh about it.*
> **Vicki, 46, executive officer, married 12 years**

Baring it all

The last of the taboos to consider is what you wear to bed – or more specifically, what you don't. There's a spectrum of bed attire that runs from neck to ankle coverage, through to underwear such as pants and singlets and on to sleeping naked.

There are many reasons people give for sleeping naked:

- a level of freedom and comfort
- responding to and managing a high natural body temperature
- not having to deal with the hassles of nightclothes becoming tangled and uncomfortable
- the feeling of skin touching the skin of a partner
- less clothing to wash
- a general commitment to being naked.

If both parties are comfortable with the practice of sleeping nude then all is well. But people who have been brought up with a certain level of modesty may find nudity in bed confronting and inappropriate. As with so many other aspects of our social being, we bring a sackful of moral and social beliefs to judge the behaviours of others. Any type of nudity can have a dramatic effect on those who were raised with the message that it is clothes on at all times of the day! Sometimes it's just that you don't like the feel of another person's skin in the same way that other people do.

> In 2002 I met my second wife, and we soon developed a very intimate relationship. She slept nude, all the time. It didn't matter if she had guests, if the kids were around, or what, when she slid into bed, she slid in naked. I questioned her on this, and to my surprise, she thought I was the one that needed enlightening. She was right!
>
> I felt uncomfortable at first, sleeping nude with her both at her house, and at mine. (I often slept over and on occasion she would sleep over with me.) But she didn't care, she wasn't going to wear anything and be uncomfortable. So I began to sleep nude, too.
>
> **Andy, 42, married for 6 years**

> I stopped sleeping naked when I was with a boyfriend, not because I didn't want to be naked, but because he almost insisted that I sleep with clothes on. I don't know what kind of message that is supposed to send, but I'm not seeing him anymore, that's for sure.
>
> **Libertine, 29, www.albertastars.com**

> Being touched by my boyfriend's floppy penis at 2 am was never romantic or sexy. The reality for me is that it affected my ability to be intimate. I found it desensitising.
>
> **Justine, 32, town planner**

That is my tour through some of the realities of bed sharing. I know the behaviours – both good and bad – discussed are not a complete list. This is because every couple is different and faces different challenges at different times in their life when it comes to why, how and who they sleep with. And it's the differences that are a critical factor in any discussion on the topic.

Each of the behaviours identified as 'bad' when it comes to sleeping with another person probably elicited responses that range from 'OMG – I totally get that and it's the reason I can't sleep with my partner' through to 'OMG, I can't believe anyone could be that petty – get over yourselves and just go to sleep'. The purpose of naming these issues is to highlight that sleeping in a bed with another person night after night is not a simple task, that is, it is not a simple task for everyone.

Some interesting facts to leave you with from the National Sleep Foundation Poll (America) 2005:

- When one spouse has a sleep problem, 75 per cent of their spouses end up with sleep problems too.
- If a spouse snores, the other spouse loses an average of 49 minutes of sleep each night.
- More than one third of people with sleep issues say the issues caused problems in their relationship.
- One quarter of spouses admitted that their sexual relationship had been affected by sleep issues.
- Twenty-three per cent of couples experiencing sleep problems end up in separate beds anyway.

PAUSE FOR THOUGHT...

🌙 Do any of the behaviours outlined in this chapter keep you from sleeping at night? For example,
- How many blankets/bedcoverings are on the bed?
- How thick or thin is the doona/duvet?
- What temperature is the room?
- Are the windows open or closed?
- Is the fan on or off?
- Is the air conditioning on or off? If it's on – what temperature?

🌙 Have you spoken to your partner about what keeps you awake?

🌙 How do you manage to get back to sleep if your partner disturbs your sleep?

🌙 Are there nights where one of you has had to find an alternative place to sleep because your partner's sleeping behaviours are keeping you awake? If so, do you have arrangements in place? What are they?

🌙 Have either of your sleeping behaviours been the cause of arguments in your relationship?

④
The decision

'There is nothing in the world so difficult as that task of making up one's mind.' – *Anthony Trollope*

Now that we've dived between the sheets of the potential pitfalls of sleeping with another person, you may be left wondering, where to from here? The answer to that question may, or may not, be quick and easy. As complex beings, we humans can surprise ourselves, and each other, with responses to unforseen issues that arise when navigating the murky depths of relationships.

For some couples, the decision to amicably sleep apart is a no-brainer. It's sensible, practical and logical, and poses no threat to the security of the relationship. For others, however, it raises deep fears that can manifest in feelings of rejection, guilt, betrayal and shame. For some, the ritual and meaning of sharing a bed is so important that if this part of their relationship is challenged, the bedroom walls start collapsing around them.

Vive la différence!

Consider any advice from this book, or from other people you may discuss the topic with, within the context of *your* circumstances, *your* own needs, *your* partner's needs and the needs of *your* relationship. These needs change, as you change, your partner changes, your life situation changes, your finances change, your career changes and ... I'm sure you get the picture. Everyone's relationship is bespoke – so make your decisions as unique as you are, and as tailor-made as haute couture.

This chapter summarises some of the key steps you can take to protect your relationship when making a difficult decision. I offer some tips along the way. These are intended to get you thinking about how you might begin to make the decision about changing your sleeping arrangements.

If you feel that raising the prospect of sleeping separately from your partner is going to cause a problem in your relationship, you need to be honest about this and decide why. For some couples, sleeping apart is a high-stakes decision – with potentially strong emotional responses to the suggestion.

To start, you might want to consider how much meaning is wrapped up in sleeping together (or apart) by you and your partner? For me and my husband, actually sleeping in the same bed every night wasn't all that important to either of us, so the meaning we attached to sleeping together was insignificant. However, the rules we created around spending time in a bed together and maintaining the rituals around goodnight and morning kisses were important because having a close physical relationship means a lot to us.

The emotion attached to the act of sleeping together each night will differ from one couple to the next. The vulnerability shown by sleeping next to another person is a sign of intimacy and great trust. So if you no longer want to sleep with your partner, are you saying that you don't trust them and you don't want to share that level of intimacy anymore? When we can't separate the emotional from the practical we run the risk of allowing fear of the unknown to develop into feelings of guilt and shame.

After knowing there are other people who sleep separately, I can finally let go of the guilt I felt about having separate rooms. I can barely function if I haven't had enough sleep and wake with a headache [that stays] for the whole day ... Some intimacy has been lost but it's better than waking up angry every day.

Des, www.mamamia.com.au

We have only been sleeping in separate rooms for six months, but I still have a bit of guilt that this will eventually tear us apart. I rationalise this by thinking if we are going to be apart, we would be apart – this wouldn't be the thing that would cause it.

Anne, 44, senior manager, married 20 years

It was hard at first as I felt guilty. But once we got into it and both felt so much better the next day after a good night's sleep, we just knew it was the right thing for us to do.

May, 66, retired, married 40 years

If sleeping separately is an issue because it negatively affects your relationship's security and stability, then it might be wise to look at that part of your relationship before making the decision to sleep separately. It's a bit like buying a ticket for the Sydney Harbour Bridge Climb before finding out if you're afraid of heights. It is a good idea to do an inventory of the foundation of trust and commitment in the relationship before you put those overalls on and climb up the hallway to the spare room.

While couples might have phases in their relationship where they take time out and sleep apart while resolving issues, sleeping apart permanently is a whole new ball game. I am not a qualified relationship expert, but I am confident that it is a good idea to have your relationship house in order before moving into the realm of separate bedrooms. Doing so will prevent the act of wanting to sleep separately from being confused with making a statement about other issues you might be dealing with together. So before you start redecorating the spare room, you might want to consider what defines relationship success for you.

All the decisions we make in life are fundamentally driven by our priorities. Often these priorities are driven by our subconscious and don't reveal themselves explicitly, but they always influence our decisions. For example, if you are resolutely determined to lose weight, you are less likely to have a hamburger for lunch because your priority is to stop eating food that is high in calories. However, if you are feeling sad and find comfort in food, you may have a hamburger because your priority is to make yourself feel better through instant gratification.

> *After a previous failed relationship (nothing to do with sleeping) I knew that without sleep I became a mess. The breakup was bitter and protracted and the lack of sleep contributed to me developing a mild clinical depression. What I did learn though was that a big priority in my life was to always sleep well. That was non-negotiable. My new partner, who I love dearly, had a steep learning curve when coming to terms with that fact that I wasn't going to compromise on getting my sleep. We spend between three to five nights apart each week, and if I need it, sometimes, more. It was a tough reveal at the beginning of the relationship, but luckily he is understanding about my situation. To be honest, he appreciates the fact that on the nights when he isn't sleeping all that well he has the space and freedom to pop his laptop open and do some work or watch a movie to pass the time until he can fall asleep again.*
>
> **Maddie, 35, health professional, married 6 years**

We had been sleeping apart one or two nights a week throughout our whole relationship, but when the first baby came along, sleeping separately every night became essential. Each of us had particular reasons for absolutely having to get some sleep. As a surgeon, when I was operating the next day I had to be well rested. The other days, Maree needed to sleep so she could function well enough to look after the baby and carry on with work. We simply took turns at sleeping in the room downstairs. It was very practical, and very necessary.

John, 33, married 3 years

Now that I've had the luxury of my own room and my own bed again, I won't be giving it up. I love shutting the bedroom door behind me and entering my own space to relax and ponder and rest. It sustains and nurtures me. There is nothing I like better than slipping into my bed each night, knowing I will sleep undisturbed until morning. Being able to spread out in a walk-in wardrobe is a definite plus as well. In time, if life does happen to bring a second partner for me, he will definitely need to be happy with a two bed/two room policy.

Veronica, 50, divorced after 25 years of marriage

So if you plan to raise the topic of sleeping apart with your partner, this could be a good time to do an audit of what your priorities are in your relationship – and find out if they are the same as your partner's. On the next page is a simple exercise to help you both determine your priorities.

Read the following statements then rate them, from YOUR perspective, in order of priority (1–10) according to how important YOU think they are to YOUR relationship. You can even consider just picking your top five priorities.

- [ ] Our relationship is viewed as successful by others.
- [ ] Letting your partner know that you love them every day is essential for a happy relationship.
- [ ] Important decisions in a relationship should always be made by both people.
- [ ] Spending quality time together every weekend is important.
- [ ] Good, regular sex is an important part of our relationship.
- [ ] There should be an equal division of domestic duties between me and my partner.
- [ ] Some form of close, physical contact with my partner every day is important.
- [ ] Agreeing on the financial aspects of our relationship is important.
- [ ] A couple should never go to bed without resolving an argument.
- [ ] A relationship should allow each person to have some space to do their own thing alone every week.

How do you think your partner would rate the statements? The same as you? Would you like to ask them to do the exercise? Then compare notes. Looking at the different ways you and your partner rate these activities might provide interesting insights for both of you.

Tip 1 – *take some time to work out the relationship priorities for you and you partner*

The connection between relationship priorities and sleeping apart is very important. If your highest priority is to be able to sleep when and how you want so you feel rested and healthy, and your partner's priority is to sleep in the same bed because that equates to a successful marriage, then you will have a tough time reaching an agreement. Many people interviewed for this book hid their separate sleeping arrangements from family and friends because a priority for them was to present as a happy, normal couple. However, other couples were open about the practice because their priority was sleeping well and what other people thought about their arrangements was not important to them.

> *I have told one person at work that we have moved to separate rooms. I will never tell my parents. Why not? The social stigma that there's something wrong if you're not sleeping together. While I find the experience liberating, I don't think I will ever get comfortable about telling people.*
> **Anne, 44, senior manager, married 20 years**

> *I'm open about it because it just works fine for us. What I care most about is sleeping enough that I can deal with my life. I know we're okay.*
> **Charlotte, 24, teacher, married 1 year**

So in your relationship, whose priorities are the right ones? Well, of course, neither and both. Our priorities are simply our priorities. If you start thinking in terms of right and wrong, it creates conflict or competition with your partner's priorities. However, these differences need to be discussed and clarified and sometimes compromise will be necessary. This doesn't necessarily mean someone has to give up their priorities – often a robust discussion and creative solutions can allow you to embrace both sets of priorities.

Another difference that affects people and can lead to conflict is having different needs. I might compromise on sleeping separately because your need for sleep is a high priority for you. However, you might compromise on telling friends we sleep separately because of my need to have this arrangement remain private. Needs also inform priorities.

Like many other topics touched on in this book, the issue of identifying, negotiating and managing priorities within your relationship can be researched through other means and is something you may want to look at, depending on your situation. Thinking about what your relationship and your personal priorities are, and how these sit alongside those of your partner, will help you to decide if separate rooms are going to be an option.

> *I moved to the spare room in our house as I could not sleep with my husband because of his snoring. He kept the main room and I think I gave him the better room as I was the one leaving the shared bed. Why did I do this? Mainly the priority for me was getting sleep. Our new house will have two main rooms – both with ensuites, that's one of our new priorities.*
>   Leanne, 41, HR executive, married 15 years

> *When I fell pregnant for the second time I knew I needed to sleep every night. I am so tired, I am asleep by 7 o'clock every night. I need my sleep and I need space so I can sleep diagonally across the bed; it's the only way I can get comfortable. He tries to sleep with me and complains there's no room, so I tell him to go to his own bed. He snores so loudly – like a tractor. I simply cannot function the next day if I sleep in the same bed as him. Maybe in the future we might be able to sleep together,*

but at the moment, getting enough sleep is my priority, so it's separate beds.

Charlotte, 24, teacher, married 1 year

Tip 2: Don't underestimate (or overestimate) the emotional response

If you haven't skipped directly to this chapter you would have realised by now that you're not alone in having trouble sharing a bed and/or a bedroom. Even though a couple may be the consummate hosts at dinner parties, spend hours together happily tending their garden or make killer bridge partners, coming together in a small space every night, when both parties are at their most vulnerable because they are tired, may prove to be one of the tougher challenges you faced as a couple.

Issues around sleeping with another person can be just one person's or they can be shared by both partners. Certainly a shared problem will make the decision to sleep separately easier, but if you are fighting the battle alone, with a partner who wants to share a bed, then the path to separate slumber will be trickier to navigate.

My husband sees my inability to sleep in the same bed (because of his snoring) as my problem. He is happy to sleep with me, but I'm not [happy to sleep with him]. I feel that there has been a negative impact on the relationship and it's seen as my fault. Over time he has come to understand how much we both value a good night's sleep though.

Amelia, 41, mother of two, married 12 years

I think he tried to take responsibility but I don't think he fully understood how it was affecting me. The underlying feeling I had was he thought I was making it up.

Louise, 48, teacher, together 7 years

> *My husband is an insomniac, has been for years (since before we met) so there's not a simple solution regarding being stressed over something in particular. He would prefer to sleep alone and there have been times when I've gone to the spare room but I hate it. To me that's housemates, not a marriage. I crave intimacy and feel rejected when he suggests I go to the spare room. He DOES love cuddling as much as me, before and after sleep, it's just the actual sleeping he'd rather do alone.*
>
> CJ, www.mamamia.com.au

How you approach a conversation about sleeping issues may differ depending on whether you are jointly or singly making the decision to sleep apart. However, what is similar in both scenarios is the initial honesty required to bring the problem out in the open.

How do you manage difficult conversations with your partner now? Is talking to each other about the tough stuff something you do easily, or does it take a crisis to bring feelings out into the open? Being honest with yourself about how you and your partner deal with high stakes decisions is an important conversation you may need to have with yourself before settling down for a 'deep and meaningful'.

As I've said, raising this topic is going to bring some emotions to the surface, no matter what the state of your relationship. Even when my husband and I were sleep deprived and coming to the realisation that we were going to have to sleep separately, making the first decision to just sleep apart during the week brought me to tears. I was scared about what this meant for our relationship as I had not thought for one minute that I would sleep separately from my partner. Were we strange? Could this work? Was it the beginning of the end after only six months? They were all valid questions at the time.

> *Years back when we first made the decision to spend some nights apart there was the question of 'Is this okay? Is it a harbinger of other problems?' But I think practicality won out at the end of the day.*
> **Neil, 46, HR executive, married 19 years**

When you have an emotionally charged discussion with your partner, do you always know how they will respond to a discussion of this nature? Can you confidently and safely predict the reaction when you give them bad news, or news that is going to adversely affect them?

The longer you have been in a relationship, the more likely you will be able to predict your reaction and the reaction of your partner to these types of conversations. However, we often surprise ourselves at our reactions to certain events and news and cannot entirely predict the emotional response we will have. Afford your partner the same flexibility. Raising this topic may be more provocative than you think. So while there is no way you can prepare for unexpected emotions and responses, being aware that the reaction might not be what you expect will at least allow you to be forewarned, if not forearmed.

Tip 3: Plan how you will communicate with your partner about your issues around sleeping together

When you decide to actually raise the issue of changing your sleeping arrangements, may I start by cautioning against launching into the topic without some planning and preparation.

At an absolute minimum, it is not a good idea to open the conversation after you have spent another night thrashing around the bed due to your partner's snoring, teeth grinding or all-night movie watching. Chances are you won't be in the best frame of mind to raise the issue. Let's face it – you may not even have the power of adult speech. Being calm and coherent is a good foundation on which to begin a discussion. So at least wait until you are well rested and in the realm of the rational.

Any marriage counsellor worth his/her qualification will tell you that solving problems in ANY relationship takes commitment, effort and a whole lot of patience, determination and good will. So when faced with the challenge of raising the issue of separate sleeping with your partner, go back to basics. The fundamentals for exploring the details of an issue are a good place to start getting your thoughts in order, so that's where we're going to start. The *how, why, when, where* and *what* of talking to your partner about sleeping separately.

How?

As a starting point, you need to consider how you and your partner communicate. A good working relationship is based on effectively communicating all the time. But are you and your partner great communicators? And to be honest, how do you know for sure?

This book is certainly not going to delve into the theory of how couples should and do communicate. There are countless books, workshops, encounter weekends and counsellors who can help you and your partner in that area. And to labour a point – because it's just so important – the way you and your partner communicate is going to be unique to you. One thing I do know from years of personal experience though is that sleeping separately requires vast amounts of communication.

I expect honesty and if my husband has a problem or issue, let's address it, talk about it and see what we can do. He has hinted that he wants us to sleep in the same room together to feel closer, but I like to sleep diagonally across the bed. We've talked about getting a king-sized bed, but then there's the issue of snoring and I don't know how we're going to get around that – it's just too much. We do talk about it. We're open and honest about how we are feeling. I try to see things from his perspective, too. So it's just a matter of having open and honest communication. I can't read his mind so he needs to feel confident telling me what he's thinking about our arrangements.

Charlotte, 24, teacher, married 1 year

When it comes to talking to your partner about changing a core tenet of your relationship, you need to be realistic. Don't set yourself up for disappointment. If having difficult conversations is not one of your strong points, then keep it simple. Don't assume you can have a deeply intimate, nurturing conversation if you've never had one before. Having a tough conversation successfully is a skill. That's why UN negotiators get paid a lot of money and consultants across the world make a fortune teaching others how to be great negotiators and have 'fierce' conversations. But I'll bet they still get it wrong sometimes with their partners because of the unpredictability of a deeply emotional relationship.

Psychology 101 tells us that most people avoid difficult conversations with loved ones (and probably lots of other people) because it makes them feel uncomfortable. Unfortunately, if you avoid dealing with a troublesome situation, you may just be prolonging the agony and building resentment. Harbouring feelings of resentment against your partner is a danger to the health of your relationship. Feeling resentful of any person's behaviours can develop into a slow-burning anger that doesn't do anyone in any relationship any favours.

> *I know that a contributing factor to the issues in our relationship is the fact that we don't talk to each other enough. We're not beyond fixing, but I get so angry that he won't talk about problems as readily as I do, and I know it's such a cliché because women want to talk more than men. He wasn't overly happy that we moved to separate rooms, but I've tried over and over again to explain to him how much better I feel now that I actually get some sleep at night. I feel guilty that he's not happy with our arrangement, but am also a bit angry and resentful that he won't give anything to me that shows he understands my situation. I read a quote recently – 'Marriage is not a noun, it's a verb. It isn't something you get, it's something you do'. So, I guess we just keep on doing this marriage and work on the newer version of what was before. I just keep saying to myself 'back to the drawing board' to find a way to show him we can make this work.*
>
> **Christine, 35, working mother, married 10 years**

When sharing a confined space with another person, resentment can build for all sorts of reasons. A common example is the friction that arises from differing approaches to routine domestic tasks. Who hasn't experienced, or caused, frustration with a partner for not taking out the garbage, not renewing the toilet roll, stacking or unstacking the dishwasher, not hanging towels up after use, leaving tissues in bed etc.

While these areas of potential conflict can be viewed as trivial, when silently fumed over and then bundled with other disparate, yet annoying behaviours and a bad day at work, we may find ourselves exploding in volcano-like proportions at the smallest of irritations, much to the bemusement of our partner, because the emotional pressure that has built up is akin to Mt Etna after a 50-year dormancy.

If your partner keeps you awake, or regularly disturbs your sleep, or interferes with how you want your bedroom's environment to be, and you don't tell them – how are they supposed to know?

> *I know I snore and am not proud of it. But I'm asleep, so how am I supposed to know what it's like to be kept awake night after night? I'm asleep, but she thinks I should understand how she feels. I'm sorry, I just don't and yelling at me doesn't actually help.*
> **Chris, 38, married 8 years**

> *During menopause my sleep became broken and increasingly elusive. While I could account for my mood swings, I thought my husband was having a phantom menopause because of his increasingly foul temper. After repeatedly questioning as to what was bothering him he finally told me (yelled actually) that he hadn't slept properly for three months because of my newly developed erratic sleeping behaviour and furnace-like temperatures. Dumbstruck and just a little p***ed off, I pointed out that this was news to me and all he had to do was speak up. I felt embarrassed, furious and helpless all at the same time. I wish he had told me in a kinder way, realising that it was uncontrollable by me and equally as annoying. He said he didn't know how to bring the subject up as he too was embarrassed. Honestly, 29 years of marriage and you would think we could get this stuff right between us.*
> **Nicola, 55, retail manage, married 29 years**

If not sleeping at night is affecting you negatively and you feel it's a problem, then, simply, it is a problem.

Some couples speak proudly of their great 'bed life' and how they just soldier on with each other's little quirks in bed because that's what good couples do. These conversations can make you think that you should try harder and learn to cope with broken sleep because other people seem to be able to do it. However, if disrupted sleep prevents you from functioning at work, and with life in general, know that it is enough of an issue to raise in your relationship.

The challenge can be trusting how you feel, clarifying these feelings for yourself, finding the words to clearly explain your situation and then working out how to articulate this to your partner in a loving way that makes them believe you. This is easy to say, but not so easy to do.

> *My husband was unhappy that I was sleeping on the couch every night. He told me he felt that we were flatmates with benefits. But his snoring and restlessness was keeping me awake every night and I couldn't function well enough to look after our children. I just sat him down to have a talk about it and showed him some bruises from where he had 'hit' me during the night and he was devastated. I knew we needed to have a purposeful conversation about the situation and I don't think you can work through an issue like this unless you have that conversation. After the talk he understood why I had made the decision, but the honest talk is needed.*
>
> Caroline, 30, photographer, married 7 years

We all like to feel valued and acknowledged by significant people in our life – especially our partner. Frustration can build when we tell another person how we feel and they don't believe us. Having concerns dismissed by another erodes trust and respect in a partnership.

If your partner does not believe that your sleep is being disrupted, you may need to find ways of clearly and calmly proving your reality. Simple tactics such as having a third party confirm your assessment of the annoying behaviour, recording a snorer, taking photographs of extreme sleeping positions, or keeping a journal of when your partner wakes you can help. If you are really desperate, you could possibly employ the devices used in the *Paranormal* movies and set up a camera. While these tactics might seem extreme, hard facts make for more productive conversations than relying on anecdotes and emotionally charged tales of woe.

> We recently shared a hotel room with a good friend to save on costs, and when said friend fell asleep and promptly began snoring, my husband was amazed that anyone could put up with it. And he thought I'd been exaggerating all these years – it was good for him to get his own medicine!
>
> **Sash, www.mamamia.com.au**

> It might sound childish, but I recorded my husband's snoring on my phone when he continued to suggest that I was exaggerating the volume and ferocity. I titled it 'The Lion Sleeps Tonight' and felt a degree of satisfaction when he was stunned into silence when watching it. Our conversations about how I couldn't get much sleep certainly changed after that.
>
> **Lulu, 42, legal professional, married 6 years**

> I decided my boyfriend needed to see the carnage caused at night from his bed acrobatics so every time I woke because the covers had been wrenched from me again, or he'd done another tumble turn and rolled on to my side of the bed, I got up, turned on the light and woke him to point out the state of him and the bed. The first night he thought it was a bit entertaining because he would just go back to sleep, but by about the fourth night, he started to get cranky with me. But it wasn't over. By night six, he agreed that being woken multiple times every night was not much fun.
>
> **Justine, 32, town planner**

While honesty – both in facts and feelings – is an important part of why you are raising this subject with your partner, don't use it as an excuse for disrespect and contempt, or as a chance to take a swipe at your partner for something else, under the guise of separate sleeping. It's true that you need to express how you feel to your partner and tell them the truth, but you also need to consider the other person's feeling when choosing your words as once you've said something – there's no taking it back. And maybe avoid an excessive use of adjectives when describing the behaviour.

Douglas Stone, Bruce Patton and Sheila Heen's book, *Difficult Conversations: How to Discuss What Matters Most*, provides insights into why people fail to communicate on difficult topics. Their book identifies three sub-conversations that take part in any difficult conversation. One of these sub-conversations – 'The "What Happened?" conversation – considers where the truth lies in a contentious issue and how agreed facts might actually mean something completely different to each party.

You will have your truth about what is happening in bed every night – as will your partner. You will also have your version of what needs to happen to address the issues you are having in bed every night – as will your partner. I am sure you have had discussions with your partner where your version of events do not match, but you are both vigorous in defence of your version as the most truthful and accurate account. Sound familiar?

Truth is an interesting concept. We all feel confident our version of life is THE truth. Unsurprisingly, our view of the world can tend to be a tad self-centred as human beings are driven by ego and a basic instinct to fight for what we believe is right. The lens that we view life through is shaped by values, morals, judgements, cultural twists and social mores. We also tend to believe that we know why other people are making choices that affect us because we try and rationalise their behaviour by thinking about what we would do in that situation. This thinking on behalf of others is a recipe for disaster.

Both of these common human behaviours can lead us on a trip down Disaster Road if we construct the contents and the outcomes of a discussion without genuinely considering the other person's input. Patton and Heen give three pointers when dealing with the 'facts' of a difficult conversation.

- *The Truth Assumption* – we often fail to question one key assumption – 'I am right, you are wrong'. There's only one hitch: I am not always right. Difficult conversations are almost never about getting the facts right. They are about conflicting perceptions, interpretations, and values. They are not about what is true, but about what is important.
- *The Intention Invention* – the error we make is simple: we assume we know the intention of others when we don't. Intentions are invisible so we make them up based on what we know.
- *The Blame Frame* – the third error we make is that most difficult conversations focus significant attention on who's to blame for the mess we're in. Talking about blame distracts us from exploring why things went wrong and how we might correct them going forward. Focusing on the conversation instead allows us to learn about the real causes of the problem and to work on a plan to correct them.

Before deciding that you know what's going wrong and then possibly how you can fix it, try to develop a curiosity about your partner's version of events so you are confident your ideas won't create an even bigger problem because you have the facts wrong. Do you even know if sleeping together is an issue for them or if it's a topic they are prepared to discuss?

Simple questions that are a good way to start a conversation include: 'How well do you think we sleep together?' or 'If you had one concern about our sleeping behaviours/patterns, what would it be?' or 'What would you say if I told you that I'm not getting enough sleep each night?'

How your partner communicates is yet another consideration you need to throw into the mix. Keep their style in mind. People feel less threatened if you can communicate in a way that is familiar and comfortable to them. If your partner likes facts, give them facts. If they want detail, tell the story. If they respond to an emotional take on the topic, then wear your heart on your sleeve. Some people just want to get straight to the solution and what it means for them, so make sure you get through to at least the end of this chapter so you can begin to articulate what it is that you want.

Thomas Bradbury and Benjamin Karney, authors of *Intimate Relationships*, make the point that in a relationship, disagreement is inevitable, but conflict is optional. This is based on a theory where strong, clear communication takes the place of blame laying, finger pointing and aggressive, thoughtless fighting. There might be times when talking about separate sleeping that you don't agree with each other or feel emotional about the topic, but avoiding a situation where you are in conflict is certainly preferable. Again, if you need more information about communicating with your partner, further reading or support from a counsellor or psychologist might be worthwhile.

Tip 4: Clearly, factually and calmly explain why your partner's behaviour is disturbing your sleep

Why?

While this might seem like an obvious question, does your partner really understand why their behaviour is disturbing your sleep? They might know that you are cranky with them in the morning because they snore, or accidentally end up with the covers on their side of the bed, but have you calmly and with sufficient detail explained the effect of their behaviour on you? What is it about their bed behaviours that interfere with your sleep at night?

I recommend you take some time to think about how you might be able to clearly articulate why you find sleeping with your partner difficult. Think about how you could explain how their behaviour affects YOU, rather than making accusations that blame them for their behaviour. The examples in the table on the next two pages might help. Remember that many annoying, nocturnal behaviours are not a choice people make. They are just part of the wonderful array of characteristics that make us all unique and are mostly unintentional.

When we know how our behaviour is affecting others, we are more inclined to change it, depending, of course, on how much we care about the other person.

If you have a partner who is inclined to be a bit less considerate or flexible, convincing them that their behaviour is impacting negatively on you and then having them care enough to change could be your particular challenge.

> *Sharing a bed just wasn't working. He would get up between 4–5 am every morning and then he would go into the ensuite bathroom and put the light on. So all the things that I didn't do to let him sleep when I came to bed later than him each night, he was just marching on and doing regardless of the fact it woke me up. Therefore resentment was building up with me and because he was the one that went to bed early, he was always in control. I would feel guilty and uncomfortable going in to the room, turning a light on and sitting up reading if he was asleep – but that type of behaviour didn't seem to bother him.*
>
> Kaye, 66, together 14 years

I have no quick or easy answer for dealing with a self-centred partner. There are many reasons why some people are less inclined to be considerate than others. My guess is that if your partner is not considering your needs in the bedroom, they are likely to be this way in other areas of your shared life.

Here are some examples of how you can reframe statements about how your partner's behaviour is affecting your sleep:

What you might feel like saying to your partner	What you might choose to say instead
Honey, your snoring is driving me insane! I can't get any sleep!	I'm such a light sleeper that your snoring keeps waking me during the night and I'm not getting enough quality sleep to function properly.
Why should I have to wear ear plugs every night so you can lie there and snore like a rhino?	Even though I can sleep through your snoring when I wear ear plugs, I can do it for a while but after about three days they irritate my ears and then I can't sleep because of the irritation.
If you steal the covers off me one more time I swear I'm going to kill you!	When you toss and turn in bed you often move the covers so much that I don't have any, and then I get cold and wake up. Because it happens a few times each night, my sleep is broken and this makes it hard for me to keep up with the kids the next day. It makes me grumpy and resentful. I don't want to feel like that, but it's what happens when I can't sleep.

What you might feel like saying to your partner	What you might choose to say instead
Stop getting up SO many times during the night, it's really, really annoying. Why can't you just go to bed and stay in bed? I can.	When you get up during the night, you disturb my sleep. I find it hard to fall back to sleep because I lie awake thinking about when you will get out of bed again.
How about you just marry your laptop/smartphone so you never have to be apart?	When you use your laptop in bed at night, the movement from you typing and the noise, even though it's not really loud, keeps me awake. I really need to get a good 7-8 hours of sleep every night so that I can think clearly at work.
WOULD YOU JUST STOP FARTING WHEN YOU ARE ASLEEP!!! DO YOU HAVE DEAD ANIMALS IN YOUR BODY?	Were you aware that the smell from your farts is so strong that it wakes me up? I get really upset and I find it hard to get back to sleep because I am so angry that I'm awake and you're still asleep.

Can you see the difference? One statement has the potential to make your partner feel bad and has a strong possibility of putting them on the defensive because they feel under attack. The other might help them understand the issue from your perspective. Simply naming the behaviour, without actually explaining the issue from your perspective and the impact it has on you, does nothing to increase your partner's understanding of your situation.

Communicating with your partner is the way to address this concern and is well outside the scope of my advice – but I do wish you well in helping them to understand that you too have rights when it comes to sleeping each night.

Tip 5: Plan when and where you will have the conversation so that your partner will be at his most receptive

When and where?

I've put when and where together as they are common bed partners in this problem-solving framework. The location of your chat may be heavily influenced by the time it takes place and vice versa – you may choose a particular time to have a conversation and this may dictate where it happens. As touched on earlier, your best bet is to raise the issue at a time when both of you are in a rational frame of mind and in a location that is conducive to a productive, adult conversation.

> *When I screamed at my husband at 2.30 am one Friday morning that I couldn't sleep with him anymore, I don't think it really had the best outcome – initially. I was having a crappy week at work, stressed trying to have a report finished for Friday afternoon, Greg [my husband] was snoring worse than normal with a cold, when he wasn't snoring he was coughing, and I just lost it. All he could talk about though was how sick he was feeling and how thoughtless I was. This made the situation worse for me and I ordered him out of the bed. We didn't talk much over the weekend and, yes, I know it wasn't the best way to raise the topic of sleeping apart. But hey, I'm human.*
>
> **Maria, 38, database analyst, married 8 years**
>
> *I had a really bad cold, was having trouble sleeping and Maria thought it was a good idea to wake me at some ridiculous time, shrieking at me for snoring or something. I told her she was*

thoughtless as it was me who was sick and I needed my sleep to get better. I get that I have to talk about stuff in our marriage, but I did suggest she could pick her times a bit better. I do remember being particularly p***ed off with her for a few days.

Greg, 39, engineer, married 8 years

Realistically, the issue of disturbed sleep is unlikely to be solved with one conversation. Consciously choosing when and where you will raise the topic is a wise move. As Greg and Maria illustrate, raising the topic when either of you is tired and not thinking rationally is not a recommended approach for success.

When buying a house your focus is location, location, location. When raising a tricky topic with your partner, focus on timing, timing, timing – and location. Be sensible and use some logic about when you bring up the topic. For example, don't try and strike up a conversation with them when they are on their way to or from work, they have just sat down to watch their favourite show on television, or they have scheduled something that you know about and the talk will keep them from getting there on time.

You know the times when your partner is at their best and worst, so maximise your chance of success and pick a time they is likely to be at their best.

Depending on their temperament, you may even choose to warn your partner that you want to have a chat about something. It may prevent them feeling ambushed, or because they were not aware you wanted to talk, arrange to be out somewhere or doing something else.

And as for the where, think carefully. If you are thinking of using a public place, for example a restaurant or a public walkway, do consider your partner's needs. If their emotional response is strong, being in a public place may make them feel defenceless and detract from the chance of getting a positive outcome from the conversation.

Lying in bed on a Saturday or Sunday morning could be precisely the time you know your partner is at their most rested and communicative. For some couples, a post-coital chat could provide the necessary intimacy to raise an issue such as this as there is often a deep feeling of trust after a couple has had sex.

I could give more examples of when and where *might* be good, but the reality is that you know the answer to these two pieces of the puzzle better than anyone. If you are reading this and thinking 'there is never a good time', then I suggest you bite the bullet, take your chances and pick what you think is possibly the time and place for you to manage the conversation to the best of your abilities and talents.

Tip 6: Be honest when considering the positives and negatives of changing your sleeping arrangements

What?

Of all the questions to prepare for, I think this is the most important: 'What do you want?'

Do you even know what you want? Are your thoughts limited to 'I just need to get some sleep every night' or have you spent a lot of time thinking about how you might re-engineer your current sleeping arrangements to make everyone's life better?

As the person raising the issue, you do have a responsibility to take the lead on what the 'new world' is going to look like. Simply saying 'I can't sleep with you' is probably going to limit the scope of your partner's response options and may also limit your opportunity to manoeuvre the conversation towards the outstanding plan you have devised to solve your sleeping troubles.

In planning to raise this issue with your partner, be very clear about what you are trying to achieve. Do you just want to open the discussion on the problems you have when you sleep with your partner? Or are you seeking to find and put in place a solution that involves changing the current sleeping arrangements? Be honest, do you just want the problem as you see it acknowledged, or are you well past that and pining for your own space every night?

Even though you might think you have all the answers and the 'best solution ever', you need to be prepared to concede that this may not be the way your partner sees it – in fact they may think it is the 'worst solution ever' – especially if they have not been involved in any of the thinking and planning for the change.

This may surprise you, but what you see as the solution to your problem is probably going to have positive and negative consequences. Just the same as staying in a bed with a person who keeps you awake all night has negative consequences, moving into another room might have some negatives too. As a rational and reasonable person, be prepared to admit to the negatives – ignoring them is foolhardy. We all know that not every decision ends in a win-win situation. It's tough, but that's life. Make sure you are clear and honest about all aspects of the decision, all plusses and minuses, as it will make for a more balanced and complete discussion.

Tip 7: Be able to describe to your partner exactly what the change to your sleeping arrangements is going to look like, what the change to your relationship is going to look like, and be open to their suggestions, too

Don't limit yourself to thinking there is only one answer to your problem/s. Depending on how your partner is disturbing you, there might be a range of options that you can suggest or that your partner might offer in reply, once you open the dialogue. And if your ultimate goal is for separate rooms, you may need to consider some interim steps along the way.

> We were both exhausted, cranky, sleep-deprived parents of two energetic boys struggling to keep up with life. We discussed sleeping in separate beds for a few days a week to catch up on sleep, and a few days turned into weekdays, then we would try to sleep together on weekends but that still didn't work so we have very happily been getting a lot more sleep and having a happier, healthier and better relationship in the years since we decided to separate – our beds, that is. We both highly recommend separate beds if your relationship is as important to you as ours was to us.
>
> Karen, www.radionational.net.au/lifematters

Admittedly, for some bed sharing incompatibilities, sleeping in a separate room might be the only option available, but get creative and be open to a range of suggestions.

Chapter seven explores the range of options as alternatives to hopping into the same bed every night, but finding the right option for you might come down to deft negotiation skills.

Your particular circumstances may require one or a combination of solutions. For example, sleeping in separate rooms three to four nights a week, and then no television on the

nights you sleep together. But whatever solution you do come to, it's really important to remember:
- don't focus on only one option as it may not be the only one (or the right one)
- get creative and investigate several options that may be available
- be prepared to try a few options – especially if your partner has suggested some.

You may even consider talking to other people about your situation as they may see a solution that you can't.

The next part of winning your partner over to the new world order is considering how the changed arrangements will affect your relationship. If your partner has a strong attachment to the practice of sleeping together every night, be prepared to describe what your relationship is going to look like – and not just the physical sleeping arrangements.

Tina B Tessina, an American psychotherapist points out that, 'Couples who choose sleeping apart need to make an extra effort to connect every day and be physically close in whatever way possible. It's already difficult for most couples to find time to discuss things, keep up to date with each other and solve problems together – three main functions of a working marriage – sleeping apart adds one more obstacle to the mix.'

If your partner foresees a loss of intimacy and physical contact as a result of sleeping apart and then equates these perceived losses the start of the end of the relationship, you need to find ways to reassure them that is not the outcome you foresee or want. What will you be able to tell your partner about the new version of your relationship that will reduce concern? Remember, just because you have something in mind, doesn't mean that your partner shouldn't have input.

Have you thought about how the loss of physical contact is going to be addressed if you move in to separate rooms?

If you think that you don't actually care about this – all you want is a good night's sleep – you may find that when you are well rested and feeling a little more in control that you do want to physically connect with your partner. This is why keeping all options and possibilities about your physical relationship uppermost in discussions is a really important part of managing this change. As many couples report that a good night's sleep rekindles their relationship, you may want to ensure that whatever you negotiate in terms of new sleeping arrangements doesn't shut the door to maintaining or improving the physical part of your relationship.

So what does your future look like in terms of sleeping arrangements? And if they are going to change dramatically, how can the physical and emotionally intimate parts of the relationship be cared for? That is up to you.

Every couple has different ways of staying connected based on what is important to them as individuals, as a couple and as a family. What you do in terms of managing your sleeping arrangements and managing your relationship to cater for those changes requires thought, planning, sensitivity, creativity and a commitment to the cause.

Tip 8: Get ready for the sex talk – be able to explain how you think sleeping separately might affect your sex life (don't forget to accentuate the potential positives)

One of the trickiest problems to tackle when raising the prospect of sleeping apart is dealing with the question of 'What is going to happen to our sex life?' This aspect is, but not exclusively, a bigger concern for men.

Dr Neil Stanley points out that, 'We are the only species that equates sex with being in bed and then falling asleep'.

And herein lies another social construct – the one that associates a successful sexual relationship with sharing a bed every night. Klösch describes the association of 'sleeping together' with 'being sexually active' and there is certainly a cultural implication that if a male and female share a bed then there is the chance of sexual activity. Stanley makes the point that 'sex and sleep are entirely separate entities, whereas we have put them into almost the same activity where if you are not sleeping next to somebody, then you are not having sex with them and that is just foolish in the extreme. It doesn't make sense.'

Because of the cultural connotations we place on 'sleeping' with another person there is often an underlying suggestion that you might 'get' or be expected to engage in sex when you hop into bed with each other. The expectation that bed equals sex puts another layer of complexity in place for those who look to their bed as a place of rest after a busy day. Stephanie Coontz suggests the idea that a person should be permanently turned on and permanently available is an unnecessary burden for modern couples. She also challenges the assumption that if you choose to sleep in another room, away from your partner, you're maybe not very sexual.

> *My sons have all said to me that if I'm not there when dad wants sex, there'll be problems. Good luck to him I say.*
> **Von, 72, married 55 years**

> *I think the issues around why people are concerned that you're not sleeping in the same bed are more about sex. If you are not sleeping with each other then other people assume you are not having sex. People feel the need (men particularly) to say they are having a lot of sex. We have a saying – 'We have full visiting rights, but then he can f*** off when he's done.'*
> **Melissa, 47, executive, married 27 years**

Most likely, you and your partner started your relationship with passionate, lustful sex where you couldn't wait for the opportunity to be in bed together. But science and sociology tell us that these lustful ways naturally wane as a relationship progresses, children come along, responsibility kicks in and we find a sexual routine that fits in around all the other 'stuff' in our lives.

Do you think that sleeping separately will affect your sex life? Are you able to articulate your thoughts about any possible effects of sleeping separately on your sex life? Can you share these with your partner? Remember, the effects might be positive.

Some couples don't feel comfortable talking about sex and think that sex should just happen naturally – no communication required to ensure that each partner is happy, satisfied and having their needs met. If this sounds like you and your partner, then moving to separate rooms to sleep may create uncertainty for you both about how sex will still happen.

So whether you plan to suggest that you would like to move out of the bedroom permanently, or just sometimes, you may want to include your sex life on the discussion agenda. Even a gentle quip about having visiting rights or 'your bed or mine' could help to put a nervous partner's mind at ease and reassure them that you can't foresee any drastic changes to the current 'sextus quo'.

On a practical level, you are probably heading into uncharted territory with this suggestion, so the truth is that you may not even know what your sex life will be like if you move to another room. (There are some suggestions in Chapter six if you want to skip ahead and get some pointers for your chat.)

Sleeping separately certainly does not mean an end to, or even an interruption to, your sex life. In fact, many couples report an improved sex life after moving to separate rooms, mainly because having sufficient sleep every night means they aren't so grumpy and tired, and as a result, they feel like sex more often. (They also feel more loving and receptive because they no longer want to physically harm their partners as a result of night after night of pent-up resentment and anger.)

This fact may be a good starting point for a discussion about why moving to separate rooms might actually improve your sex life.

A number of women report that having their own space means that they don't feel like they are 'on tap' all the time for sex with their partners. In discussing this issue in her book, *A Strange Stirring*, Stephanie Coontz reported that several women spoke of the pressure to always be in the same bed was bad for their sex life because it made sex sort of routine, instead of making the choice and an effort to initiate it. The outcome of sleeping separately may be that sex becomes more exciting because it's not just a matter of 'Oh, you're there, so let's do it' but more sought after and deliberate.

> *My husband and I have an intentional intimacy now. Moving to separate rooms after being together for 24 years has actually made our sex life more exciting – it's removed the obligation of just going to bed and finding each other. Now we visit the other's room and it feels more special.*
> **Anne, 44, senior manager, married 20 years**

> *Because we both get a good night's sleep, we argue less because we have the patience to work through our problems better than we used to. Because of this we seem to have become more tactile with each other and simply, this has led to more sex. We're not doing it all the time, but I would definitely say we have more sex than we were having, say, about four years ago.*
> **Mike, 52, landscape gardener, married 23 years**

Bed's not the only place to have sex. I would feel like I'm from the 1950s if I went to bed every night and just expected that sex was going to happen. Sleeping separately certainly stops the '2 ams' and I no longer have to deal with the 'tap on the shoulder'. But we have a very active sex life. I'm happy and I know he's happy.

Amelia, 41, mother of two, married 12 years

There is an increasing number of couples embracing the concept of date nights, and there is no reason why this can't continue through to arranging a romantic tryst with your partner where you invite them to your room on Friday or Saturday night for a 'date night with benefits'.

Realistically, when it comes to sex – depending on the level of importance placed on it by you and your partner – sleeping separately could prove to be just what you are looking for to give your sex life a shot in the arm, rather than it sounding the death knell to this part for your relationship.

I hope this chapter has provided you with a simple framework to organise your thoughts and plan a strategy to have a discussion with your partner about your sleeping issues. Having tough conversations with anyone isn't easy. Humans like to protect those close to us and that protection extends to emotional safety. If you can find the right words to say at the right time, you may find that potential hurt is minimised and you can achieve a much-needed level of honesty.

Now let's see what the outcome of your discussions might look like as a negotiated agreement.

Tip Sheet Summary

Tip 1 Take some time to work out the relationship priorities for both you and you partner.

Tip 2 Don't underestimate (or overestimate) the emotional response.

Tip 3 Think about and plan for how you will communicate with your partner about your issues.

Tip 4 Clearly, factually and calmly explain why your partner's behaviour is disturbing your sleep.

Tip 5 Plan when and where you will have the conversation so that your partner will be at his most receptive.

Tip 6 Be honest when considering the positives and negatives of changing your sleeping arrangements.

Tip 7 Be able to describe to your partner exactly what the change to your sleeping arrangements is going to look like, what the change to your relationship is going to look like, and be open to his suggestions too.

Tip 8 Get ready for the sex talk – be able to explain how you think sleeping separately might affect your sex life (don't forget to accentuate the potential positives).

> **PAUSE FOR THOUGHT...**
>
> - How well do you and your partner communicate with each other?
>
> - Do you ever discuss how (not if) you communicate?
>
> - Have you and your partner talked about what your sleeping issues are and how they could be resolved?
>
> - How do you and your partner communicate about your sex life?
>
> - What happens in your 'home' when one person wants something the other doesn't? How do you let each know what you want?
>
> - If you know you aren't great communicators and have unresolved problems in your relationship, have you ever considered seeking external help to assist you to communicate better?

⑤

Negotiating the outcome

> 'Everything is negotiable. Whether or not the negotiation is easy is another thing.' – *Carrie Fisher*

Once you feel you have covered the how, why, when, where and what of bed sharing, then you need to prepare for the outcome of your discussions. Are you and your partner able to negotiate a mutually acceptable decision about changed sleeping arrangements that you can both live with? Take a deep breath and begin.

If you both agree that your sleeping arrangements need to change, consider yourself fortunate. And if you can agree immediately on how the new arrangements will work, then bravo! The ability of couples to find solutions to tough problems is dependent on a vast array of variables and managing those variables will no doubt remain a great source of income for psychologists and self-help authors for years to come.

As noted, it's tough to hear someone else's view of, or solution to, a problem when you know you have the answer. It's even tougher when the other person doesn't see how fantastic your solution is and has the audacity to challenge, pull apart or even refuse to agree with your insightful and well-crafted plan. When they do come up with an alternative or fail to agree to your brilliance, what are you going to do?

As mentioned earlier, a component of problem solving for couples is having and then exhibiting goodwill. But what exactly does that mean? Words and phrases used to explain goodwill include benevolence, kindness, friendliness, cheerful acquiescence, consent and a favourably disposed attitude towards. They all mean the one thing – playing nice while agreeing to something you may not necessarily want to agree to. Ow! Negotiation hurts!

Having goodwill is a state of mind. It's a willingness to enter into something with your best manners, your best attitude, your nicest words and a healthy dose of care and concern for the other person with whom you are negotiating. This care and concern needs to centre on finding an outcome that works for them as well as you, so that it really is the best outcome.

> *I think my husband understood I could no longer physically sleep next to him. He has mentioned a few times that he misses me. He sleeps better when I am next to him; he can go back to sleep better when I am next to him. When he asked if we could ever sleep together again, I said, 'If you can do something about your snoring, then maybe we can' – but I would not expect him to go through the operations needed to fix the snoring. Three of them didn't work for my mother. How did I feel when he said that? Nostalgic, because I knew it would never happen. Quite honestly, I can't sleep next to a log cabin being built with logs being sawn all night.*
>
> **Suzette, 40, administrative assistant, married 17 years**

There is much that has been researched and written about the outcomes and purpose of negotiation. Business and diplomatic negotiations have serious terms such as 'distributive', 'integrative', 'interdependence', 'leverage' and 'strategic'. While negotiating with your partner need not involve the high-level theoretical knowledge and skills of a UN diplomat, there are aspects of formal negotiation that are worth considering.

Two notions are particularly useful: 'Negotiation is the principal way that people redefine an old relationship that is not working to their satisfaction' and 'The goal of negotiation is not to win, it is to succeed'. Both of these are precisely what you are aiming for – a successfully redefined relationship.

As humans, our fundamental survival instinct keeps us bound to our self-interest, and appropriately so. This practice served us well in our early days of fending off wild animals and foraging for food in the pursuit of basic survival. So it's natural that we continue to manoeuvre and arrange our lives to meet our own needs. But when we have to accommodate other people who don't have exactly the same plans that we do, then we have to find ways of manoeuvring to keep as much of our planned outcome as we can.

To help you negotiate with your partner to change your sleeping arrangements, I offer three potential strategies. I'm going to offer them in the order of least favourable to most likely to succeed. They are sacrifice, compromise, and consensus.

Sacrifice

In this book, I am using sacrifice in the context of when one person gives up something important or valuable so that another person can have something else. Just wanted to clarify that, in case anyone thought I might be suggesting the ritual killing of another human – in this case for the crime of keeping you awake for five nights in a row by snoring loudly. A very important distinction.

All close and long-term relationships require a degree of sacrifice. It's a behaviour that oils the wheels of marriages, friendships, work relationships and parenting. In fact, many people might see sacrifice as the ultimate expression of love for another person and sometimes it is. When we give up something we want, e.g., to eat Thai takeaway instead of pizza, we do so because we are invested in a relationship and understand that part of socialising successfully in that relationship involves not always getting what we want. It's inevitable that in a relationship we have to make some sacrifices – unless we are outrageously rich and famous and can demand compliance from our minions – and most of us are happy to forgo what we want to keep someone we care about happy. But we all have our limits.

In their article 'Giving Up and Giving In: The Costs and Benefits of Daily Sacrifice in Intimate Relationships' Emily Impett et al look at two competing values in Western society – one that emphasises an ethic of altruism, selflessness and sacrifice, and the other that emphasises individualism, autonomy and a relentless pursuit of personal freedom. They make the point that in our intimate relationships, we often find ourselves at a crossroads having to choose between these two paths – giving selflessly to a romantic partner or being true to our own wishes and desires.

For example: a husband has a season ticket for a particular sport that he attends every week. It's an event he loves because he catches up with friends. On request from his wife, he happily stays home from one weekend's game to look after the children so that his wife can meet a friend who has unexpectedly arrived in town. The husband may feel great satisfaction knowing that he has cared for and responded to his wife in a loving manner. This type of sacrifice moves the husband towards a desired end-state and is called an *approach motive*. In this scenario, there is no resentment as the husband willingly gave up his needs for his wife. In contrast, what would happen if the wife had asked her husband to stay home four times during the season, despite knowing the importance of this social activity to her husband and then became very angry and aggressive if he said no? If the husband agrees to stay home to avoid angering his wife or having an argument over the request, he is likely to feel resentment or other negative emotions that detract from his satisfaction in the relationship. This type of sacrifice motivates the husband to avoid an undesired end-state and is called an *avoidance motive*.

Research has shown that sabotaging or constantly denying your own true wishes and desires in a relationship is associated with increased psychological distress and decreased relationship satisfaction. Impett et al found that those people who sacrificed something because they wanted to avoid an undesirable outcome experienced more negative emotions, lower satisfaction with life, less positive relationship wellbeing, and more relationship conflict. Not a good list of outcomes for anyone, or any relationship.

On the other hand, social psychologists have investigated the positive role sacrifice can play in relationships. There are a variety of demonstrated relational benefits, including increased satisfaction and a greater likelihood of persistence over time to work on overcoming issues. However, findings highlight that it's the motivation for the sacrifice that determines if it will be healthy for the relationship.

Simply put, if your motive for sacrifice is to be loving towards another then you are more likely to experience a positive outcome, but if your motive is to avoid conflict, the long-term outcomes will be negative, driven by resentment.

So what are the wrong reasons to sacrifice your needs for someone else's?

A sacrifice that is motivated by avoidance is going to cause issues in the long run. Conflict avoidance is the main driver for many people who sacrifice their own needs. It might be easier to put up with the snoring than to have a big argument with a partner who resolutely believes a couple should sleep together.

Another misguided motive for sacrifice is the belief that by sacrificing something you want, you will show your partner how much you care for them. You may have had the conversation to explain what is disturbing your sleep, but your partner told you that they just want to be 'close to you' every night, so you continue to endure disturbed sleep to show how much you love them. You may even believe that by sacrificing your own needs, you are providing a good example that your partner will emulate in the future. You may harbour a silent expectation that they will start showing you how much they care for you in return with a sacrifice or two of their own (but they have no idea about this expectation – because you haven't told them). Noble behaviour, but probably futile, and certainly unhealthy.

While the above explains behaviours with seemingly good intentions, it's the motivation behind the sacrifice that makes it unsustainable. If you are left feeling annoyed that you haven't been true to yourself by agreeing to stay in bed with your partner, or you feel that you made the decision to stay there because of an imbalance in power, then I would suggest you consider why you continue to sacrifice your own needs for your partner's needs. Think about what this type of behaviour is achieving in the present and where it is leading as you head into the future.

Yet another misguided reason we sacrifice our needs is to use the sacrifice as a bargaining tool in a future transaction. For example, 'I'll give up my movie night with the girls to go to your last-minute work function if you come to Bill's birthday party with me next week instead of playing golf'. While we have all used this tactic on occasion, if it's an ongoing behaviour in your relationship, it might be time to consider how healthy the dynamics of the relationship are.

Sacrificing your own comfort, pleasure, needs and health for someone else might make you eligible for sainthood, but it's a negotiating technique that relies on an uneven power balance and a degree of disappointment for one person in the relationship. If every time you want pizza you give in and have Thai takeaway to please your partner, I would suggest your partner is not considering your needs and wants. In the long run, is this what you want?

> *Moving to separate rooms was a big plus for us. I was getting to the point where I was really resenting him carrying on with his preferred lifestyle and I was feeling I just had to go along with it. So now, I am doing what I want to do and I'm more relaxed. Resentment has been taken out of the equation. I think it's definitely had a beneficial effect.*
>
> **Kaye, 66, together 14 years**

If you always agree to have the bedroom temperature at 19°C while you shiver under the sheets, or you give in every night and allow your partner to watch television into the early hours of the morning while you can't sleep, and as a result you are unhappy and resentful and sleep deprived, then you aren't being true to yourself or your relationship. If, in finding a solution to your sleeping issues, either of you sacrifices something very important when you don't really want to in order to avoid conflict, the outcome is again neither sustainable nor beneficial to the relationship. It's not easy.

> *After a year of Greg's snoring getting worse, I decided to start sleeping on the couch in the lounge room. I slept there for about two years. He knew it was happening but beyond a couple of yelling matches, we only had a bit of a vague, grumbly chat about it. I thought he would offer to go to the couch sometimes or offer to do something about his snoring so I could sleep properly in our*

bed. Why did I keep doing it? I thought month after month he would see the sacrifice I was making and step up to do something about it. It became a bit of a test I set him – even to see if he would say something, or ask me why I was sleeping out there or if I was getting any sleep. Why didn't I force him to go to the couch? I think I didn't want to hear 'no' as an answer and I really just thought he would do the right thing after seeing what I had done so I could sleep. You think you're leading by example, but in this case it was my own fault for not speaking up. I'm sure friends probably thought I was being a bit of a martyr and I guess I was. It's separate rooms now though. We finally sorted ourselves out and had a talk about it. I did work it out.

Maria, 38, database analyst, married 8 years

If you look honestly at your motives for either staying in a disrupted sleeping environment or moving to an alternative sleeping arrangement, and you find that the decision involved a sacrifice you didn't want to make, then it might be back to the drawing board to find another solution that will be longer lasting, fairer for both of you and better for your relationship.

Compromise

The next level of negotiated outcome is when you and you partner compromise on alternative sleeping arrangements. What's the difference between sacrifice and compromise?

Sacrifice is when one person completely lets go of something they consider valuable to allow another person to continue to have or do something they want, but the other person does not change at all. Compromise is when you both agree to give up something in exchange for a concession or new behaviour from the other person.

Compromise has greater longevity than sacrifice as a negotiation tool because both parties agree to do (or not do) something for an improved joint outcome. When you are both emotionally or physically invested in a solution there is a greater chance of success. Compromise still has an element of sacrifice to it as it involves an element of giving up or giving away something as it is a settlement of differences through mutual concession. The major difference is that both parties are motivated to commit to some type of change in order to work towards a perceived improvement.

A compromise might be as simple as one person in a couple who wants to sleep together every night agreeing to let the disturbed sleeper have two nights a week alone in the spare room.

While sacrifice has a win lose framework, compromise is a little further along the spectrum towards a win win agreement. However, many argue that because you are both giving something up, it is actually lose lose – neither of you gets what you really want. That is relationships though – there is always a need for give and take.

> *Living with someone is definitely a compromise situation. After 37 years, we decided that we have a spare bed and whoever feels that they are lacking in a good night sleep can use the spare bed. I always stay up later than my husband (I watch TV or read). He gets up early in the morning (and sneaks out to not wake me).*
> **Kate, www.mamamia.com.au**

> *After the first night I spent with my now husband, he was such a terrible sleeper I told my friends there was no way I could even consider him as a possible boyfriend! To compromise, we now spend maybe two nights per week sleeping apart so we can catch up on sleep and spend the other nights together.*
> **Anonymous, www.mamamia.com**

> *I felt guilty about keeping the light on as it kept him awake. He is such a kind person and considerate of me, so I was happy to turn the light off and not read to be considerate towards him.*
> **Elizabeth, 60, married 25 years**

> *Did we have any feelings of guilt about moving to separate rooms? No. You just get used to it and accept it. You don't expect the other person to be perfect. It's just part of the compromise of being married and putting up with each other's foibles.*
> **Anthony, 62, education professional, married 25 years**

In my early thirties, one of my closest friends and I were single for a few years. We put the time to good use endlessly discussing our single status and the awesome guys who were going to come along, sweep us off our feet and give us the 'happy ever after' we so obviously deserved. One of the topics we spoke about often was compromising in relationships. Our main uncertainty was around just how much you had to compromise to make a relationship work. After my friend met her awesome guy and settled down, she told me she had worked it out – 'If you are asking yourself, "Am I compromising too much?", then you are'. Those words have stuck with me all these years, and I have shared them with friends who have found themselves with the same dilemma to give them the 'aha' moment I enjoyed. It's an easy test, and one that has served me well, and not only in romantic relationships.

When negotiating a compromise it's important to be clear about what you can and can't accept. This goes back to strong, clear communication. Finding the best compromise may not be one conversation away: it might be twenty discussions away.

> *My husband and I periodically slept separately, mainly if we were a bit upset with each other. We would always end up back in our room together eventually. After one particular*

time he left our room after an argument, I thought really, this is absolutely heaven. No snoring, I could have the room as I wanted it with the window open when I wanted it and I slept undisturbed by his blanket stealing and restless sleeping. I still asked him to come back in though as I wanted to do the right thing. But when he had been back in for two days I thought I don't want him in here, I don't want to compromise anymore. I found that so liberating.

Anne, 44, senior manager, married 20 years

About eleven years ago I started not being able to sleep because of my husband's snoring. At first I would watch a movie on the laptop to drown him out, but that still meant I couldn't sleep. He's also very restless and will sometimes hit me, not on purpose though. Because we don't have a spare room in the house I just sleep on the couch now. It's the only way we are going to stay married because if I had to sleep in the bed with him we would be divorced. I just have a pillow and blanket in the lounge room. I'm used to it and I get a much better night's sleep out there. It's not a failure of our relationship, it's what works for us. It's what works for me.

Caroline, 30, photographer, married 7 years

Compromise involves change. The industry that has evolved around managing change in humans is enormous. Counsellors, mentors and self-help gurus recognise the resistance we have to change. We like our lives to be predictable and when they aren't, we get 'out of whack', don't know what to do and may even start acting out because we are unhappy with the new circumstances in which we find ourselves.

In the context of sleeping, we get used to sleeping on the same side of the bed, sleeping in the same position, with the same pillows and blankets, and in some cases, with the same person next to us. When all our certainty and comfort is challenged, we are likely to feel threatened and defensive and fight to keep what we know, if only because we know it. Keep in mind that with change comes the chance to have a new arrangement that may be even better than what we had before – we just didn't know it at the time.

Aside from one person moving out of the bed, there are other types of compromises that can take place for bedtime incompatibilities. Solutions such as a person who is disturbed by the light of a reading partner using an eye mask, or the reading partner using an eReader instead of a real book (and a real light), do involve changing our behaviour, but they are a small compromises. Other compromises may be bigger.

> *While not being a huge fan of every technology fad that comes along, I love the iPad. My husband can now read at night without the light having to be on and without the 'swoosh' of the pages turning. He's not allowed to listen to or watch anything on it. It's a good compromise for me needing quiet and a darker room and him wanting to read. Mind you, if it doesn't continue to work, then it's back to the drawing board.*
> **Nicola, 55, retail manager**

> *If I can't sleep I need to read and this can sometimes be for a few hours. In those cases, it's me who gets up and goes to the spare room. I know Ann can't sleep if the light is on so it's not fair to her to do that. Also, if one of us is travelling for work the next day, then the other one has to go to the spare room. This lets the person travelling have access to clothes and the bathroom early in the morning without having to worry about waking the other one. We manage sleeping with a very practical approach.*
> **Neil, 46, HR executive, married 19 years**

> *Our kids are sleeping worse than ever now and this means that we take turns sleeping between our main room and our spare*

room. We normally do this night about, but it depends what we have on the next day work-wise. We both want to feel able to cope as much as we can so this means we need to sleep apart and alternate the good night's sleep with the broken sleep that comes with looking after the children. For me, I don't sleep all that well anyway – and it's getting worse – so having the peace and quiet of the room downstairs means I have a better chance of getting a good night's sleep.

Maree, 30, health professional, married 3 years

What will be useful as you work towards finding a compromise is taking the time to really understand your partner's point of view on the situation. If you can take the leap and 'sleep between their sheets' your understanding of what they are agreeing to commit to in the compromise may be more real to you and easier to fit into the context of what you are going to do or give up doing.

Consensus

The third and most successful outcome of a negotiation is reaching consensus.

While compromise still has traces of sacrifice, in that you both make concessions to come to a solution, consensus is defined as 'a solidarity in sentiment and belief', and 'agreement between all the people involved' – for our purposes, all two of you. It's when you can both honestly say, 'I believe this is the best decision we can arrive at for us at this time. I will support what we need to do to make it happen.'

Some argue that a consensus has an element of 'heart' involved over and above the 'head' factor required for compromising. It's when you and your partner can consider all the factors involved in the issue at hand – and that involves each other's perspectives – and come to a decision that you both agree is a solution. A consensus implies a genuine commitment to the decision because both of you have listened to the other's needs and your shared interests have been met. What you have actually done is looked at the bigger picture of what each of you need in regard to sleep, considered what's important for both of you and agreed on a new way of 'doing' sleeping at night.

In his book *Consensus Through Conversation*, Larry Dressler highlights why consensus is the most logical and sensible approach to decision making and recommends it when the decision:

- is high-stakes
- has the potential to fragment those involved if made poorly
- involves a solution that will be impossible to implement without strong support and cooperation from those who must implement it
- has no single person who has ultimate authority to make the decision
- has no single person with all the knowledge required to make the decision
- has people with a stake in the decision having very different perspectives that need to be brought together
- needs a creative solution to address a complex problem.

Although *Consensus Through Conversation* is aimed at a corporate audience, all these descriptors perfectly fit the challenge faced by a couple who can't immediately find a solution that will address the issue of one or both of them experiencing sleepless nights.

If you are thinking that there is a grey area between compromise and consensus, you are right. Consensus involves both of you making changes to your sleeping arrangements. However, it is the attitude towards, and the motivation behind, the decision that takes you from compromise to consensus. It comes down to how you approach the task of finding a solution to the problem and how you accept the solution once it's been agreed upon.

A compromise may see you or your partner holding on to your position, for example, 'I feel like more of a couple when my husband sleeps next to me every night' – but agreeing to behave in a way that doesn't match this. And yet you do it willingly with no resentment, no 'if only ...' thoughts. Consensus is about finding a way to shift your thinking, and therefore your position, and work with your partner to find the best solution for both of you.

Most importantly, reaching consensus means that in coming to the decision, neither of you feels that your position on the matter is misunderstood or wasn't heard.

> *After sleeping apart for a few days, then a few weeks at a time, one night my wife and I just agreed that the struggle to share a bed wasn't worth it anymore. I resisted the decision most and didn't think I would ever agree to a permanent arrangement of separate rooms. But in the big picture of our lives it worked best for everyone. I felt a sense of relief, and funnily, really close to her. I still miss having her in the bed every night, but enjoy the times in the early morning when I slip into her bed and share a few hours cuddling her. I don't think I will ever feel comfortable talking about our separate sleeping arrangement as I think a husband and wife should share a bed, but my snoring was just too loud. I would rather have my wife, who sleeps in a separate bed rather than not have my wife.*
> **Wayne, 41, married 18 years**

> *After 30 years of marriage and many variations on our sleeping arrangements, sleeping apart was just so convenient for us both. We are in the same house, we still see each other, there are as many conjugal visits as either of us wants and we both get what we want from a bedroom. In the big picture it makes so*

> *much sense. If he wants to come and spend a night he can, but he knows that it can't happen too often! He knows his snoring disturbs me and he cares enough about me to let me sleep. We've accepted that this is our sleeping life.*
>
> **Brooke, 52, educational professional, married 30 years**

In trying to reach consensus, you may find a solution that you hadn't thought of before. Consensus involves a degree of 'I have my way of thinking about something but I could be wrong. So I am going to listen to you and allow my mind to be influenced by you. I may not fully agree but hopefully by sharing and listening we can agree to a new solution that is ours.' It is an attitude fuelled by goodwill. Remember goodwill?

And while this all sounds warm and fuzzy and oh so easy, the reality is that it isn't always. If your partner is adamant that you both stay in the same bed because that's what couples do and all you want to do is move into another room because you cannot bear one more hour, let alone night, of their restless legs, then it's going to be tough to find a solution that meets such disparate needs.

Consensus takes time and work. It all depends where you are coming from and where you are going to. The further apart the positions, the bigger the challenge. This is where you return to the basics of communication and continue to in the hope of finding that elusive and hallowed common ground that just hasn't revealed itself yet.

Humans have an interesting capacity to hear something and go away and ruminate. If a seed of a solution is planted, then the germination time might be a bit longer than you hope, but may still take place. So you may have to sit tight, revisit the topic and not give up. Onwards and upwards – always.

Can't get to yes?

After you and your partner have demonstrated outstanding communication skills, and you've both showered each other in boundless goodwill to find a solution to your sleeping issues, then what next? We'll get to that in the next couple of chapters. First, I want to talk about what happens when you don't reach agreement.

Sometimes the best laid plans don't turn out as expected. Sometimes it's not until the twenty-fourth revision that you manage to get it right. You both need to retain flexibility while you determine what works for you, and keep talking. Don't stop talking. If you haven't been great communicators in the past, this could be a chance for both of you to hone your skills and rediscover a genuine interest in each other.

Be honest with each other about what is working and what is not. There is a chance that you will have adjustments to make that create tension and friction as you iron out the details, but honesty and strong communication should help you over any rough patches.

What if all your attempts at trying to renegotiate your sleeping arrangements don't work? Even with all the will and best intentions in the world, you and your partner may not be able to find a solution that suits you both, and that is a tough place to be.

John Gottman, psychologist and researcher who runs *The Love Lab*, says that he can predict how long a couple will last, not by studying how well a couple gets along, but by studying how well a couple doesn't get along. He notes that a relationship is only as strong as its weakest moments; these surface when a couple faces tough challenges.

As hard as it is to accept, some problems don't have solutions. The reality for some couples is that sleeping issues may cause, or be a big contributor to the end of a relationship.

> *My relationship ended because my partner could not accept that I wanted to sleep in a separate room. No matter how much I explained the substantial impact on my health from not sleeping, he would sit on the chair in the bedroom and say 'we've got to get this right because if we don't get it right the relationship's finished'. His mother had dealt with her inability to sleep by taking sleeping pills, and he was set in his ways about what a traditional relationship looked like – two people sharing a bed. I tried to explain that our relationship didn't need to end just because I needed to sleep in a bed by myself every night. A couple of weeks after I told him I was moving into a separate room, our relationship ended.*
>
> **Louise, 48, teacher**

If you can't find a solution with your partner to your sleeping issues, the best advice that I can give is to keep trying. By this I don't mean keep trying the same thing over and over again. That just makes you eligible for insanity by Albert Einstein's definition: 'Doing the same thing over and over again and expecting a different result'. But you also need to remember Winston Churchill's equally worthy advice: 'Never, never, never, give up'.

If your solution isn't working, you will need to try something different, such as:

- Finding people you know who sleep apart (there's lots out there once you start asking around) that your partner would trust and ask them how they make it work.

- Trying different ways of finding out your partner's motivations for staying in the same bed and working to ease their fears that the practice threatens your relationship.

- Finding a less dramatic solution than moving to separate rooms by suggesting small adjustments to your partner

thereby letting them work through the change in a way that is not as confronting.
- Making sure the topic doesn't disappear off your relationship radar by continuing to make reference to it or taking the chance to talk about the effects of sleep deprivation, etc. (this may be interpreted as nagging, but it is all in the delivery).

If all your efforts do not bring about a successful resolution that both of you can live with, you may need to consider external help in the form of a counsellor. Whatever you do, if it's really important to you, don't give up.

> **PAUSE FOR THOUGHT...**
>
> - Have you ever analysed the process you follow to resolve conflict, and if you have, does it work or could it do with some improvements?
> - Is one of you more of a peacemaker than the other?
> - Is one of you more inclined to sacrifice your needs for the other?
> - What happens when you come to an impasse on other issues? How do you resolve these situations?
> - Can you think of a situation where you have reached a compromise or consensus? What did that look like for both of you and how did you get there?
> - Are you individually, or as a couple, capable of talking to other people – parents or friends – to see if they have solutions you can't see?
> - Would you consider seeking help from a counsellor to work through issues that you are not able to resolve yourselves?

⑥

How to make sleeping separately work

> The best laid schemes o' mice an' men
> Often go awry
> And leave us nothing but grief and pain
> For promised joy. – *Robert Burns (1785)*

We all love that spine-tingling moment when a wave of brilliance arrives to resolve a problem and we make a plan. We organise our resources, rally the troops, communicate the plan to all involved and remind ourselves why we rule the world and are masters of our destiny.

The tricky thing about a plan is that it's just that – a plan; a proposed and sometimes inaccurate prediction about how something will be in the future. A plan is a course of action you think will bring about an intended and hopefully beneficial outcome. But life is unpredictable, and worse still, so are the other people whose help you often need to execute your plan. How many great plans have you made that have been ruined by bad weather, a late bus, a lost friend or a person who cancels on you at the last minute?

Still, our indefatigable spirit means that we never stop making plans, which is good. If we did stop, we would never solve problems, launch into exhilarating adventures or go to fantastic dinner parties with friends.

Once you and your partner decide that your sleeping arrangements need to change, then it's time for you both to put your heads down and plan. German philosopher Immanuel Kant said: 'The best way to predict the future is to invent it. Planning is bringing the future into the present so that you can do something about it now.' Planning gives you a sense of control by working towards making the unknown known. The question is: what is your plan and what factors do you include when sitting down to decide the fate of your slumbering future?

For some couples a change in sleeping arrangements just happens. An unspoken understanding that sees one person move to another room because of disturbed sleep results in a permanent move that is never discussed or formally agreed. Even though some couples are able to work within the framework of an unspoken agreement, such arrangements can be a *Titanic* heading out to sea.

> *When my husband started sleeping in the lounge room, it just kind of happened. He liked watching sport on TV, so would often sleep on a mattress in the lounge as I didn't like TV in the bedroom. There was no discussion; it was just convenient for both of us. When the kids left home he moved into his own bedroom, where he now has a TV. We weren't upset about the arrangement, so I guess we didn't feel like we had to talk about it. We talk about a lot of other things in our marriage, but just didn't talk about sleeping separately.*
>
> **Brooke, 52, educational consultant, married 30 years**

> *The decision to sleep apart happened gradually. We lasted one year in a bed together after we were married, but even in that first year his snoring was so loud, I would regularly disappear during the night to another room. Over time, I started disappearing more and more during the night, but he was such a heavy sleeper that he didn't notice. There was no*

specific discussion where we sat down, but I think there was an understanding about why I was leaving.

Leanne, 41, HR executive, married 15 years

One day it dawned on me that he hadn't come to bed for quite a few months. He wasn't cold-shouldering me and there was no attitude, but I realised we weren't sleeping together anymore. There was no specific discussion, but we did have a conversation one day that unless his snoring stopped, we would probably never sleep together again.

Suzette, 40, administrative assistant, married 17 years

We never made a formal decision to sleep separately. How it went was I would sleep at his place sometimes when we weren't living together and then he would learn that I got grumpy after not sleeping that well. Then I would kind of do both when we were living together but did have my own room when we first got a place together. I definitely slept in the same bed more frequently back then because I wanted to show I was trying but the quality of sleep never improved. Now, I try less because we have a child, are so much busier and the sleep quality is that much more important. I definitely think formally discussing it is the way to go because there are a lot of emotions around it that keep continuing when you don't talk about it directly. If you just do it at the beginning and have a plan, there is less negative emotion. For instance, whenever we would get into a big argument about something, my husband would bring this up and then I would feel crummy all over again. 'You haven't been trying; etc.' because we never defined the parameters to begin with. If you leave things 'open' then there is miscommunication and misunderstanding and a whole wack of negative emotions that come with it. So therefore, I would far more prefer some negative emotion up front but a concrete plan/decision that is worked on in the beginning.

    Christine, 35, working mother, married 10 years

I know that if my husband and I hadn't talked about the decision to sleep separately, I would have had a hundred questions floating around in my head. And in the absence of answers from him, I would have made them up. Even though I knew that sleeping together wasn't an option for us, I still needed to know answers to some practical questions when we moved to our separate rooms, such as:

- Would he still want to kiss and cuddle me?
- Would we still have a sex life?
- How did he feel about sleeping separately to me?
- How would we tell people about our decision?
- Could either of us go to the other person's bed if we wanted?

I also needed some fairly silly questions answered too:

- Would he miss me at night?
- Would he think less of me or our relationship because we were in different rooms?

I'm not very composed when I have unanswered questions hovering in my mind. I don't mind answers I might not like, but I much prefer an answer that is 'no' to no answer at all. Left alone, my brain is too creative and often errs on the negative.

    Planning to change your sleeping arrangements can range from having a quick, light-hearted and amicable chat, to a deep and confronting discussion that lasts for hours (or days) through to documenting your decisions so you have something to refer back to if details are forgotten in the future. The nature and seriousness of the discussion and planning will depend on how you best like to work when making joint decisions. If your plan is very detailed, capturing it on paper is a good idea. This can help avoid the 'but remember you said you would move to the spare room if you woke me two times in a row, not three' type of arguments. I would recommend that if there are metrics or a level of detail in what you are planning, then as a minimum, jot a few points down that you both agree to – but refrain from having it witnessed by a court officer!

If you are making a purposeful decision to change your sleeping arrangements, even a brief discussion will help create the space to bring in the changes. It will alert both you and your partner to the fact that life in bed is going to be different, and might avoid the situation where one of you feels as though the other has engaged in a covert operation designed to un-nerve or un-hinge you through deceptive bedtime behaviour. Whether planning a brief discussion or a major diplomatic offensive, remember the framework from Chapter four and answer the questions how, why, when, where and what.

Also, as discussed in Chapter four, it is a wise idea to consider a range of options when deciding how your sleeping arrangements are going to change. There are many variations of the theme of sleeping apart and although having completely separate bedrooms is as far away from sleeping together as you can get (without heading to separate houses), there are many possibilities between these two ends of the spectrum.

Importantly, be open to the likelihood that the first change you make to your sleeping arrangements may not be the last. Like many facets of your relationship, sleeping arrangements evolve over time and may need tweaking and tuning to get them right.

Klösch says that 'sleeping as a pair is not a fixed system that has to remain constant for years or decades once it has been established .... sleeping is a dynamic process influenced by many different factors such as age, gender, degree of stress, day of the week and even weather conditions'. In itself, the process of ageing and maturing precipitates ongoing change. There are few people who have the same haircut or wear the same fashion as they sported a decade ago. So just as you accept that low-slung jeans or skimpy tops no longer flatter your developing midsection, decisions you make now about sleeping arrangements may not suit you in a year or a decade's time. What's great about being a grown-up is that we can change our minds and try new things all the time – with the cooperation of and in consultation with our partner, of course.

When you begin your planning phase, be mindful of the emotional responses that talking about the changes such as nightly separation might have on you. If you are up to it, name your emotions as they surface, both positive and negative. Ask your partner how he is feeling as you talk about your plans. For example, 'I think I'm going to feel really sad and a bit guilty the first night I go to bed in the spare room. How do you think you will feel?' or 'I appreciate and am grateful that you understand how I feel about not having the TV on in the bedroom, and I know you are giving up something you really enjoy so I can sleep better'.

The suggestions I make are by no means comprehensive. Hopefully some of them might be what you are looking for, while others might spark an idea for a solution to your particular sleeping problem.

To clarify what I mean by 'alternative sleeping arrangements', I mean an alternative to a traditional couple's sleeping arrangement where most resources in the main bedroom are shared, and both of you climb into the same bed every night, share bedding, and wake up together every morning.

I group the range of alternative sleeping arrangements under three headings:

- The paddling pool
- The wading pool
- Diving into the deep end.

The paddling pool

Offering solutions that don't actually involve either of you moving to a separate room might seem contrary to the spirit of this book, but, if you are at the stage where you and your partner don't need to, or cannot bear the thought of, sleeping in separate rooms, there are steps you can take that allow you to splash around in the paddling pool of alternative sleeping arrangements. Depending on what your particular bedroom issues are, you may start to find relief for your ills by changing some of the physical aspects of your bedroom or the behavioural aspects of the people who sleep in it.

Just remember that separate sleeping is not for everyone – but getting a good night's sleep is.

Even making small changes to your current sleeping and bedroom behaviours may pave the way towards a better night's sleep.

Bedtime stories

In the battle of 'the bed readers vs the bed sleepers', there are a number of behavioural and environmental changes you can make that will let both of you have your needs met.

- The person who likes to read could stay in the lounge to read rather than reading in bed.
- You could negotiate a specific amount of time for reading in bed – e.g. half an hour.

- The reader could buy an e-Reader to minimise the noise from turning pages and, if light from the eReader is a problem, negotiate a level of brightness you can both live with.
- The reader could buy a book light that fits directly over the book to minimise light in the room.
- One or both of you could investigate bedside lights that give a more directed beam of light.
- The sleeper could wear on an eye mask until the reader is ready to turn the light out.

Oh, my boyfriend and I have had some fun negotiating this one. I absolutely must read before I sleep, and if the book is good I can read for a couple of hours before I even know it. He insists that the bedside light has to be off so he can sleep, so I've settled on reading by candlelight. I have a candle in a big hurricane lamp, which works fine for me. It actually feels sort of cozy, especially in winter. The trick of course is to be sure to blow it out before you fall asleep!
Rohanna, 25, student

One word – Kindle. All the fighting, all the tossing and turning and 'humphing' disappeared in an instant. It was a miracle.
Lisa, 45, mother of two, married 25 years

Little lamps and eye masks don't work for my husband or me. Either we both stay awake with lights on in bed, or we both sleep with lights off in bed. If one of us can't sleep and the other one must sleep, then the one who can't sleep leaves the bedroom. When we're at a motel, I sit in the bathroom to read.
Elaine, 48, married 22 years

Old bed, hard bed, soft bed ... new bed?

The age and suitability of the bed you share may be the cause of your sleeping problems. If you have been sleeping on the same old mattress, on the same old frame for a long, long time, you might benefit from an upgrade. A number of factors can impact on mattress comfort for couples and differing needs in style and firmness of mattresses become more common as people age.

Bad backs, hips, shoulders and necks can legitimately lead to couples needing mattresses that have different levels of firmness. The most common way to solve this is to change your bed to one that accommodates two different levels of firmness. This could be one mattress with differing levels of firmness on each side, or two single beds that can be put together to form one king size bed. A quick search on the internet will provide you with the information you need. This solution may see you heading to the manchester department to purchase new bed linen, so dust off your credit card in preparation.

If you have to deal with a restless sleeper, you may need a new mattress that minimises the impact of their movement on you. Latex mattresses offer this feature and might be just what you are looking for. Again, a couple of hours on the internet might prove to be an enlightening experience. If you prefer face-to-face research, a discussion about your sleep issues with a bed salesperson will update you on the possibilities that are available.

Maybe you just need to just consider a bigger bed? Two couples I know – both in their mid-forties – still sleep in double beds. I am amazed that they are able to find the comfort necessary to sleep each night, but they do and speak fondly of enjoying their cosy environment. Many couples find that by moving to a king size, or super king-sized bed, they have enough space to escape a heavy breathing or restless partner. This size of bed also accommodates those who like to exercise creativity in their sleeping positions throughout the night. If you have ever slept in a super king-sized bed, you will know that the challenge is sometimes finding the other person, rather than being disturbed by them.

> Recently we purchased a king-size bed. It's great and the tossing, turning and snoring are not so bad now. I am sure it's due to the extra space under the covers. I find it also romantic reaching out whilst under the covers of a big bed and touching and caressing the one I love. My husband agrees.
> MM, www.radionational.com.au/lifematters

Temperature tantrums

Research shows that the ideal temperature range for sleeping differs widely for each person. The wide fluctuations mean that there is no prescribed best room temperature to produce optimal sleep patterns. We simply sleep best at the temperature that feels most comfortable to each of us – just the same as some of us enjoy living in the tropics and some of us love arctic climates. (Another question to add to your speed-dating checklist.)

That said, extreme temperatures in sleeping environments do disrupt sleep. REM sleep, which we know is one of the important deep sleep phases, is more sensitive to temperature-related disruption. For example, in very cold temperatures, we can be entirely deprived of REM sleep. So a complaint about being too hot or too cold to sleep is legitimate. What can you do?

If the temperature difference is minor, you can investigate doonas that are weighted differently on each side. Similarly, having separate doonas, blankets and sheets will allow each of you to sleep at your ideal temperature.

> Having central heating in the house means that my wife is able to have the bedroom quite warm. When I then have to sleep under a thick doona, I end up throwing it off every night, but then wake up periodically a little chilly, then hot again after the

doona goes back on, then hot, etc etc. I could have slapped myself across the back of the head for not thinking of separate doonas sooner. Such an obvious and simple solution. Now I just have to get her to turn the TV off.

Francis, 37, engineer, married 7 years

I have always slept with my sheets tucked in so was frequently annoyed when my husband insisted on having his feet out every night to sleep as he complained the bed was too warm and having his feet out regulated his temperature. He would even do it in winter. I know it probably sounds very petty, but it annoyed me to think that the sheets were untucked on the other side of the bed and I would sometimes lie awake and think about it. After discussing it with a sympathetic friend, I cut all our sheets up the middle to half way and now wrap the side in the middle of the bed round my feet. Problem solved. I'm really quite normal otherwise.

Milly, 52, married 30 years

Fans and air conditioner are areas of potentially tough negotiation. When one person can't sleep with a fan or air conditioner on, and the other can't sleep without it, it is a very difficult situation. Consensus may be impossible, compromise is likely to leave both parties still giving up something they may actually need to sleep properly and sacrifice, well, we know where that ends.

Some problems don't have a solution. A number of people I interviewed cited extreme temperature differences as the cause of sleeping separate. No paddling pool for them.

Bedtime

If you have issues around what time you go to bed at night and get up in the morning, you may need to give your creativity a good work out in devising solutions around how you to avoid waking each other up. As we know that forcing a change on your body clock is not going to work, you may have to accept that this is going to be a long-term challenge.

Some suggestions to get you going:

- Lay rugs or runners on a wooden floor to help to minimise the disturbance of a noisy walker.
- Agree that when the lark heads off to bed, the owl gets ready as well, but doesn't actually go to bed until later.
- Use a low-illumination night light for the owl's convenience when they do come to bed.
- Agree that the lark's gear for the next day will be readily available in another part of the house, so no raking through the wardrobe and drawers takes place in the morning.

Would you stop that!

As we discussed in chapter three, there is a range of annoying behaviours that you can try to limit through intervention if you want to sleep together, such as snoring, stealing sheets and blankets, using laptops, watching television, grinding teeth and breathing noisily.

For example, agree on such arrangements as:

- After the first/second/third/nth time that your partner's snoring wakes you, you are allowed to wake them to change position (irrespective of whether they agrees they were snoring or not).
- If retrieving your stolen sheets wakes the 'thief', then that's the price they have to pay for taking them in the first place.
- If your partner has moved such that their breathing or teeth grinding wakes you, you are allowed to do what is needed to make them roll away to minimise the noise.

This story from the *Wall Street Journal* may provide you with a workable process...

> Rochelle Thomas has gotten so fed up with her husband's snoring over the years that she's created a 'three strikes rule.' Each time he wakes her up with his snorts, honks or shudders – shaking the mattress 'like a cheap motel-bed vibrator' – she gives him a penalty.
> Strike one: A nudge.
> Strike two: A shove or kick.
> Strike three: He's out – of the bed and down the hall to the guest room.
> 'It prevents anger in the morning from lack of sleep,' says Ms. Thomas, a sales representative from La Mirada, Calif. 'And I think it just may have saved his life, because I am sure I would have killed him by now.'

Similarly, if one of you has needs that impact on the other because you are getting out of bed at times or with frequency that disturbs the other's sleep, then alternative arrangements might minimise the disruption – depending on the facilities in your house:

- If your partner's use of the ensuite toilet at night-time wakes you, ask them to use another toilet.
- If you have only one toilet in the house and it's so close to the room that its use during the night wakes the sleeper, agree not to turn the lights on or flush the toilet if it is used just for urinating.
- If one of you has to get up early for work, or sport, or anything, then all clothes, accessories, etc. that are needed are taken out the night before and put somewhere else in the house, and another bathroom (if available) is used to get ready.

- If one of you is always later to bed than the other, then lights are not turned on and the ensuite is not used for teeth cleaning or before-bed toileting (again, if another bathroom is available).

When it comes to appliances in the bedroom, there needs to be some give and take if you want to continue sharing a bed. My best suggestion is that times for use are negotiated. For example, television viewing only until 11 pm, laptop used only for 30 minutes after going to bed. This will definitely be a situation of compromise, so all the best on this particular negotiation.

Miscellany

There are a number of other practical solutions for the parade of bedroom problems. Here are some suggestions for dealing with some of the other issues we have identified.

- If one person is bothered by a partner who prefers to sleep in the nude, then the nude partner is not allowed to touch the clothes wearer during the night unless permission is granted; if nude sleepers want to cuddle, they need to consider wearing PJs.
- If one partner cannot sleep if there is light in the room, invest in a comfortable and effective eye mask.
- If noise is keeping one partner awake, investigate the range of earplugs on the market or look into purchasing a white-noise or sound machine to create a constant background distraction.
- If eating is leaving mess in the bed and the bedroom, agree that only certain types of food be allowed in the room and that a 'no plates in the bedroom' rule applies so all dishes must go back to the kitchen before lights out.

- If children in the bed are squeezing one or both of you out, take some time to re-negotiate boundaries with your children and/or spouse about sleeping and bedrooms.
- If pets are causing a nightly exodus, you can invest in a pet bed for the bedroom.
- If the occasional illness is an issue, for example, during cold and 'flu season, pre-negotiate an agreement that one of you will temporarily relocate for a period of time, so you don't have to try to negotiate such matters at 2 am.

The suggestions above are in no way exhaustive, but hopefully provide some examples of what might be negotiated to address common disturbances. Your particular situation may require a variation on one of the above suggestions. If your dilemma is not specifically answered, I hope there is something in this chapter that gets your creative juices flowing. I don't have, and nor do I think there is, a silver bullet for everyone's unique sleeping dilemma.

The priority is to focus on a solution and not the problem, keep talking and don't limit your thinking to the obvious. Ask yourself this question: 'What needs to be different to make this work?' and revisit the idea of brainstorming solutions. The most sensible idea might come out of the most ridiculous suggestion.

If none of these ideas sound like the solution you are after, or you have come back to the book because you have tried several solutions but still aren't getting the night's sleep you know you deserve, then it might be time to graduate from the paddling pool to the wading pool.

The wading pool

If you know that you are unable to spend every night in the same bed and/or same room as your partner then there are a number of options to investigate. Again, keeping an open mind and thinking outside the box will help you find the answer to your problems.

Many couples find the answer to sleeplessness comes in the form of having semi-permanent arrangements to sleep apart. These types of arrangements are very common for couples that realise they have an issue sleeping together that cannot be resolved, but still want to spend some nights in bed together when it suits them. They like the idea of sharing a common bedroom, but value and need their sleep enough to sleep apart sometimes. How often this part-time arrangement is used, of course, depends on the issues and needs of each couple.

Some of these arrangements could be:

- Agreeing to sleep in the spare room sometimes – you can negotiate the number of times you use the spare room option, who goes to the spare room and the reasons why one of you goes there.

- If there is no spare room available, have a mattress (comfortable and pre-made) available in another room such as a study or children's room for nights when separation is needed.

- Buy a sofa bed for a study or sunroom and make sure it is pre-made and ready for full- or part-night use.

- If the situation is desperate, agree on a set of circumstances that might lead to one of you sleeping on the couch sometimes. If this happens often enough, have a set of bed linen (pillow, sheet, duvet/blanket) ready and easily accessible for the bedroom refugee to take to the couch.

Another advantage of using a spare room for occasional sleeping is the continuing relationship that is maintained within the main bedroom. This relationship allows couples to keep connected using the main room as a base and just sleep elsewhere. Some might argue this is semantic – but try telling that to the couples who have found their sleeping nirvana in this arrangement.

> *We call our spare room the 'sleep sanctuary'. Whoever really needs to sleep is allowed to spend the night there. Juggling careers and two young children means that there are months when we don't sleep together in the bed in our room because one of us is in the 'sleep sanctuary', but we choose sleep over being in the same bed at this point in our lives. If we are on holidays then we have no issue being in the same bed – but when it's our normal life, sleep is essential.*
> **Maree, 30, health professional, married 3 years**

> *We have a spare room that one of us will sleep in maybe 2–3 times a week. Often the discussion about who will sleep there happens just before we go to bed. If he is travelling I find out what time he is getting up and I will decide to go to the other bed if it's going to be so early that it will disturb my sleep.*
>
> *We mainly start in the same bed each night if one of us isn't travelling. But if I can't sleep – which happens a bit – I like to read. This disturbs Ann, so I get up and go to the spare room. It takes the pressure off both of us and we both sleep better. It's simply a practical solution that lets us get the sleep we need to deal with life.*
> **Ann and Neil, both 46, HR executives, married 19 years**

> *I only started using the spare room to sleep when I read an article about it at the beginning of the year. Neither of us had thought about it before – we just thought it was a traditional thing to sleep with each other every night. We both sleep so much better in separate rooms; it's definitely been of benefit to both of us. But where I sleep is still just the spare room – I haven't slept between the sheets yet, just under the doona cover and on*

the top sheet. My pyjamas are still under the pillow of our bed in our room, I get ready for bed every night in our room and I walk right past a bathroom to use the ensuite in our room. Our bedroom is still a part of me, I just don't sleep there every night anymore.

Elizabeth, 60, married 25 years

Another arrangement that might work for couples that are dealing with a restless partner is having separate beds in the same room. Depending on the size of your bedroom and available funds, it could be feasible to have two double beds, or two super-single beds in the same room. Hopping in to your partner's bed for a quick cuddle will certainly be easier and night time and morning chats will be unhindered.

If you know that you are neither a paddler nor a wader because you have tried some of these fixes with no success, or you just know that it's time to make the break and have your own room, then let's look at what's involved in diving in to the deep end and really sleeping apart.

Diving in to the deep end

Explaining the technical part of this arrangement is easy. You and your partner sleep separately every night.

In the deep end, you and your partner have completely separate rooms, or one of you sleeps in a different part of the house every night, but you still share the amenities of the main bedroom.

Sleeping apart permanently comes to some couples slowly. A traditional – or normal – start to a relationship or marriage sees most couples sharing a bed quite happily, but factors such as snoring, illness, children or changing priorities see them deciding at some point that separate rooms are the best.

We started sleeping together at the beginning of the marriage, but he was younger, thinner and didn't snore as loudly. Right from the beginning I did need ear plugs though. He comes from a family of snorers and his parents have slept separately for the last 25 years.

Suzette, 40, administrative assistant, married 17 years

We slept together for quite a while at the beginning. Doug started falling asleep on the couch, and I tended to leave him there as his snoring was getting worse and if I woke him and made him come through to bed, I would be the one who was kept awake because of his snoring. This lasted until about four years ago when we finally agreed that separate rooms were the best arrangement for us.

Penny, 40, mother, married 14 years

In the beginning, we were very old fashioned and 'didn't do that' (sleep apart). I started working in the bedding department of Myer in the 1980s and was shocked to find out that married couples slept in separate beds. I thought there must have been a problem in their marriage. But over the last 15 years, I started to snore, John's hearing became very delicate and he started to not sleep as deeply. I also like listening to the radio when I go to bed and that would drive him mad. I tried a few things to stop my snoring, like making a band out of t-shirt ribbing that I put around my jaw, but nothing worked and we were getting less and less sleep. You have to adapt as you change and get older, so I shifted to the spare room.

May, 66, retired, married 40 years

Margaret started working night shifts, so she was getting home at about 2 am, but not being ready for bed until about 4.30 am. This meant she would wake me up about an hour before I would normally get up. I know she was complaining that I

> would thrash around in the bed a lot – she says I'm 'theatrical in bed' – and apparently I snore. Anyway, I was losing sleep because of her sleep patterns so a few years ago we agreed that it would be best if she moved to the bedroom downstairs. We're both very happy with the decision.
>
> **John, 58, building contractor, married 30 years**

> For us, we ended up in separate rooms for a few reasons. Probably because I had a lot of surgery, then he got his knee operated on and I thought I deserved a bit of room to myself. After I had spent some time in a bedroom by myself because of my surgery, I realised how good it was having your own space. There was no going back. When we have to share a bed now it's awful.
>
> **Von, 72, married 55 years**

For other couples the decision to sleep apart happens pretty darn quickly, though this is less common than those who find it becomes a necessity over time.

> Michael and I met at 14, married six years later and have never been able to sleep together. We thought we would just get married and start sleeping with each other – but it didn't happen. We tried to sleep in the same bed, but one of us always ended up in the spare bed. We were both reasonably relaxed about it right from the beginning. It never caused a big issue for us. The bigger issue was the frustration of not being able to sleep so the decision to finally have separate rooms was liberating.
>
> **Melissa, 47, executive, married 27 years**

If your planning leads you to decide that you are moving to separate sleeping then there are a number of sub-plans that need to be made.

Where are you going to sleep?

If there is an available spare room in your house then you are set. The question you have to address is who is moving to the spare room? This one might be tricky if the bedroom you currently share is bigger, has an ensuite, has air-conditioning, has all the closet space, favourite furniture, etc. How are you going to decide who moves and who gets to stay? Flip a coin? Paper-scissors-rock? It could prove to be a tough decision.

My husband's bedroom is much larger than mine and has an ensuite. It's certainly the pick of the two bedrooms, but I prefer my room because of its positioning to catch the night-time breezes in summer and I did not want to give them up – so we had an easy task negotiating who slept where.

If one of you is more eager to move to another room than the other, then that person may find they are the one taking the less-well-appointed room, but this is not a given. It's all about negotiating what's best for both of you, given your own particular circumstances.

For couples who have children or extended families, a spare room is a rare commodity. This creates a substantial problem that needs to be factored into any plans. This particular challenge is most commonly solved by the use of the humble, but trusty, couch.

After my time sleeping on the couch we decided that I would permanently move to a separate room. Unfortunately there was only a small spare room towards the back of the house, near the kitchen. As much as I hated to admit it, I knew that that's where I was going, because I was the one making all the fuss about Greg keeping me from sleeping. However, I am very happy to say that after a bit of whinging on my part, we renovated the room, which involved investing in some good carpet and a very quiet reverse-cycle air conditioner. I have a great bed, even though it's just a double, with very nice bed linen. And when I need a glass of water in the night, it's just a short walk.

Maria, 38, database analyst, married 8 years

When we came to the agreement that we were no longer going to be able to share a bed successfully, we figured it was easier for him to just stay sleeping on the couch. We don't have a spare room because we have children and a house that just fits us all, so we bought a really comfortable couch that he can totally stretch out on and sleep. It's a proper single-bed-sized couch and that was our compromise. The good thing is that this is only a temporary solution as we are building another room for him next year. Seeing as he has the most trouble getting to, and staying asleep, being on the couch means that he can watch TV when he wakes at night.

Suzette, 40, administrative assistant, married 17 years

I have been with my husband for 13 years, but for the past 11, we have had trouble sharing a bed. Because of space problems in the house due to number of people vs number of rooms, I sleep on the couch. Sleeping there doesn't affect my health, a lack of sleep does though. It happened over time. I got sick to death of getting out of bed and going to the couch, so now I just have a pillow and blanket out there all the time.

Caroline, 30, photographer, married 7 years

Re-negotiating the romance

This section may also be relevant to those who are in the wading pool, but wading in deeper and deeper and spending more nights apart than together. Keeping connected to your partner through intimate behaviour is important when you aren't sleeping in the same bed every night. It's what makes your relationship different to the other relationships in your life. As I have mentioned a number of times, I am not talking just about sex. While that's important, it's the smaller acts of intimacy that can be forgotten or put in the too-hard basket when you don't have the daily chance to connect emotionally, socially and physically in bed together.

Dr Timothy Sharp, Clinical and Coaching Psychologist and founder of the Happiness Institute, says that couples should think about the constructs of intimacy as it relates to them as a couple. He emphasises that intimacy and sleep are separate. 'It's important to understand the separation, and then it's important to think what intimacy actually is for you. Intimacy can occur at different levels, and in many different ways. Yes, part of intimacy is sexual intercourse, and other physical acts, but they can be done in many locations at any time of the day. Then there are other parts of intimacy, hugging, holding hands, kissing, that can also be done at any time of the day and anywhere. I would encourage couples to define intimacy as broadly as possible and not limit it to just sex in bed at night. Intimacy can be whatever you want it to be, in different ways and different times. If you choose to sleep separately it does not mean you have not chosen to be intimate.'

On the flip side though, just because you move to separate rooms does not mean you suddenly have to become a couple who kisses and cuddles every time you see each other in the kitchen. What is most important is that neither of you feels as though you have lost too much intimacy because of the sleeping choices you have made.

Dr Barbara Bartlik, a New York psychiatrist and sex therapist, has identified the three greatest challenges couples face when they decide to sleep apart. While recognising that 'sleeping soundly benefits people on all levels, mind and body, and directly contributes to a longer and happier life', she also make the point that couples in this situation should 'institute strategies and rituals focused on keeping them connected romantically rather than just living together as companionable housemates'.

Dr Bartlik's challenges and solutions are:

- **Less loving touch:** Even when couples aren't accustomed to holding one another all night long, a lot of touching goes on while falling asleep and during the night. Whether intentional or not, touch enhances intimacy. It also has a measurable biological effect, stimulating oxytocin, the hormone that promotes a sense of bonding.
  The solution: Dr Bartlik urges couples to make a concerted effort to stay touchy-feely during the day. Don't just walk by each other—stop for a casual kiss or a loving pat. Hold hands on the couch, and cuddle while you watch TV.
- **No opportunity for pillow talk:** You may have lots of focused conversations about the children, the car and the dog, but there's something uniquely intimate in the kind of pillow talk that meanders here and there as you're relaxing and readying yourself to doze off at night or as you awaken and get set to take on the day. Good marriages thrive on these private, unplanned, and uninterrupted conversations.
  The solution – a hybrid arrangement: Dr Bartlik suggests trying to fall asleep in the same bed but with the agreement that if one partner's night-time habits interrupt the other's sleep, it's perfectly okay for him/her to slip off to go sleep in a different room – then toward morning, the one who

wakes up first can slip into bed with the other to share those close first few minutes of your day.
- **Fewer sexual interludes:** Not surprisingly, diminished sexual intimacy is the greatest concern people have about sleeping apart, but Dr Bartlik says that she knows many couples whose sex lives are enhanced by separate rooms – it can even lead to greater desire! This makes sense for several reasons: research shows that being sleep-deprived lowers testosterone in both men and women, which interferes with sexual desire for both genders and also makes it harder for men to have an erection and women to achieve orgasm. In Dr Bartlik's view, this is a bigger threat to intimacy than just the fact of sleeping separately. And there's also the fact that absence can, indeed, make the heart – and other body parts – grow fonder. You know what I mean.

The solution: Getting more rest will almost certainly help boost your libido. Therefore, she suggests that couples that sleep apart should make a special point of having sex regularly. If the idea of a scheduled 'date night' sounds unromantic to you, why not approach it in a way that adds sizzle to your sex life? Try to establish romantic rituals that bring you close, such as sending sexy notes to each other, lighting candles for dinner or taking a bath together. You can also make a point of engaging in pleasurable but not sexual activities that include touch such as dancing, sensual massages or simply holding hands on after-dinner walks.

I have included the detail of Dr Bartlik's advice as it captures the three most common issues and three most common solutions that most couples interviewed for this book talked about. When a couple is sleeping separately purely because they need to sleep, there is usually a strong desire to ensure the physicality of the relationship is not lost.

Most nights (and I do mean most) I will go to Fraser's room after he has gone to bed and have a chat, lie on the bed with him and at a minimum, give him a kiss and a cuddle before he goes to sleep. We sleep with our bedroom doors open so when we are both in our beds and one of us is turning off the light to go to sleep, that person will call out 'night, night honey, love you' and the response is 'night, night honey, love you too'. When Fraser is dressed in the morning he comes through and wakes me with a morning kiss and often on the weekend, one of us will wake and go through to the other's bed for a snoozy cuddle. We seek cuddles and kisses from each other often, and our sex life is healthy and not confined to the bedroom. Would we be having more sex if we slept together? We'll never know, but neither of us feels that we are missing out. We did make the effort to talk about how we would maintain physicality and intimacy when we made the decision to move to separate rooms and from time to time, we will remind each other if we feel one of us is backsliding on our deal.

Maintaining intimacy is an area where couples I interviewed spoke enthusiastically about 'keeping romance alive' and I can honestly say that no-one saw sleeping separately as a reason for less sex. Busy lives, children, stress and getting older were all cited as reasons for a reduction in cuddling, kissing and sex, but as noted in the last chapter, most interviewees felt the intimate part of their relationship benefited from being more rested. Stephanie Coontz, director of public education for the Council of Contemporary Families in Chicago, said many couples are 'confident enough that they have a nice marriage, but they don't particularly like sleeping in the same room. I don't think it says anything about their sex lives.'

Couples do speak of a need to be more explicit about their actions and behaviour to ensure the full spectrum of intimate behaviours in their relationship are kept alive, but again, the most common tales told are of positive results.

There are two parts to plan for – maintaining the intimacy and maintaining the sex. I think the best way to give examples of what can be done is to hear from the couples who have already worked it out.

Maintaining the intimacy

For us, we are naturally close to each other and maintain this by really strong communication. It's a fundamental connection for us. We would feel more distant when we haven't had the opportunity to check in with each other each day. That's more important than a good night or good morning kiss. Not that they don't happen. We try to have family dinners when we are home, which starts the conversation, once the kids are in bed it's our time to reconnect; 'download the day' with each other. We might watch TV or just sit with a glass of wine and swap stories. We are lucky that we work in the same office so often drive to and from work together, and that time adds to when we connect with each other. We definitely don't feel that we are missing out on any physical closeness by not spending every night in bed together.

Neil, HR professional, 46, married 19 years

When I go to bed, I want to sleep. But if I go to bed early enough, my husband will come and tuck me in, we sit for 20 mins and we chat and snuggle. If I wake up early, like 5 am, I will go and have a snuggle with him on the couch. We cuddle during the day, or when we're watching TV I'll put my head on his lap.

Suzette, 40, administrative assistant, married 17 years

It's important that each night before we go to sleep we spend at least an hour in bed together before one of us goes off to the spare room to sleep. Some of the time will be doing something alone, the other half will be doing something together like watching part of a movie or a TV show. Sometimes Maree will 'nag' me to make sure this happens, but it's nice to be forced to do it – I actually appreciate that she does insist on it because I think I would miss it otherwise. We also have a double shower that we use together each night. We love standing in there chatting, catching up on the day, discussing things we need to – it's one of our 'alone time' things that we really enjoy. It's downtime away from the kids and life.

John, 33, medical professional, married 3 years

Each night we sit and have a glass of warm milk together at the kitchen table and talk about the day before we go up to our beds. We head off to bed at the same time and get up at the same time. We do spend a bit of time together because we are a team and we rely on each other.

May and John, both 66, retired, married 40 years

On the weekend Doug comes into my room and we spend hours in the bed together and that's when we catch up on the week because we are so busy. Even though we will speak to each other about four times a day during the week, it's still good lying next to each other and chatting. We have human touch, but it's not overly romantic – that's just not us – but it happens and it's important. We laugh a lot together and that's really important. I'll sometimes send a text message to Doug in his bed that I would like a cup of coffee. He makes it and comes in to my room and hops into bed. It's great. Most times on the weekend we end up with everyone in the bed, me, Doug and the three children. We really do love it.

Penny, 40, mother, married 14 years

One of the things we found really important is snuggling in bed together in the morning, not necessarily for sex. That whole snuggling up, waking up, chatting in bed – that closeness of being together in the morning is really important. Particularly on holidays, we make an effort then to wander in to the other one's room at 5 am to have that waking up time together. All this is time together. It's not about sleeping together. It's about being together when the sun's coming up in the morning and you are having a natter together about the world.

Melissa, 47, executive, married 27 years

For me it's about cuddling. It's clichéd and girly, but I don't care. My partner has realised that I need to cuddle, to have the physical contact we miss out on by not sleeping in the same bed anymore. I ask him for cuddles and sidle up to him on the couch. He knows now that sitting on the couch to watch TV = cuddles of some type. I think there's some link to a primal need for touch? I'm a tactile girl so I seek to have that need met often. My partner tells me that he often hopes the cuddles will lead to more, and sometimes they do.

Justine, 32, town planner

Maintaining the sex

Sex? If you want it, it's still there. If you need it, it's still there. If you want closeness, you can ask. If I want 'company' I'll ask my husband to sleep with me and that's fine – but it doesn't have to happen every night thank goodness.

Dianne, 52, education professional, married 30 years

Having not slept together for ten years we have perfected sex on the couch. Even though we recently went back to sleeping together when the children stayed in their beds for a while, the couch still got a good work out.

Michael and Liza, 41 and 39, married 10 years

Sleeping apart has had absolutely no impact on our sex life. Having children certainly has, but we've gone from having daily sex to weekly at a minimum. And the sex happens wherever and whenever.

Caroline, 30, photographer, married 7 years

While we are not the best at talking about it, our sex life hasn't suffered. Since we've been sleeping apart we've managed to have two children – so I think that means it's okay. I still shower in the ensuite of the main room so am often in there and things just happen. I would say that in some capacity, whether we use words or not, we both know when the other would like to have sex. For us it's mostly demonstrated through actions towards each other. Sometimes one or the other will go out of their way to appear when the other is going to bed and then spend time together in the bed. I guess you sometimes have to make an effort to make it happen. Our arrangement is working well for both of us. I think that even if we were in the same bed, the amount of sex would be the same because we have such different sleeping patterns.

Leanne, 41, HR executive, married 15 years

Maintaining intimacy in any long term relationship is difficult. Let's face it, the fizz definitely fizzles after a while! Since spending more and more nights sleeping separately my husband and I too had to find our new kind of normal; a normal that is unique to us. For us it all comes down to one word: 'effort'. And not just making an effort once or twice or even a dozen times, for us it is about doing what we can every single day to keep that passion alive and keep it on track.

Like anything in life that is fabulous and worth fighting for we made the decision to openly and honestly discuss how our sleeping dynamics were detrimentally affecting our intimate time. We realised that like everything else in our lives, for example getting fit and eating right or planning an amazing holiday, we have to make an effort and put time into actively thinking about our sex life. We have to make time to put some music on and sit on the lounge together with a glass of wine. I have to make the effort to wear that sexy little nightie I know he likes when he comes home. He has to make the effort to leave me sweet, naughty notes. Or if he really wants to surprise me, and this is going to sound crazy I know, but for me to come home from work to a house that is spic and span and all the housework done is an amazing aphrodisiac. I have to say that of everything he does for me, this is a real turn on because it means he is giving me the gift of downtime and that means we have more time to relax together. This is priceless and it doesn't cost a thing, just 'effort'.

We both need to do these things; not all the time but often enough to keep things exciting yet not so often things become routine, stale and boring again. I know all these things sound clichéd but they are clichéd for a reason ... because they work. At the end of the day, we've realised that regardless of what bed we are sleeping in if we want to keep our love life and our marriage alive for many years to come then it all comes down to the effort we put in.

Emily, 30, international flight attendant, married 1 year

As for sex, well there's certainly not that spontaneity any more, but with three children, there probably wouldn't be anyway. But after having no sleep and waking up resenting the other person there's definitely not going to be any spontaneity anyway. We're more likely to have sex now because I don't actually hate Doug anymore for keeping me awake. We've got pregnant since we moved to separate rooms, so I can guarantee you we've done it at least once. I believe that women with children are much more approachable in the morning than in the evening because of being so exhausted by everything you have to do. I am so appreciative that I can fall into bed and not have my husband throw his hand on my boob. But I am equally appreciative when he slips into my bed after I have had a good night's sleep.

Penny, 40, mother of three, married 10 years

There has been no impact on our sex life at all. Whoever is keener just goes into the other's room. If you can't sleep and the other person is awake then you can go in there. It's really about being respectful of the other person. We've always been happy with our sex life, we still are but if one person wanted more then they ask the other. No problems.

Richard, 48, IT engineer, married 20 years

We still have sex, early at night because I can't stay up late. We've done the dinner, the bath, put our son to bed and then we spend time together, watching TV or reading, or we'll just lie down and talk. We are still intimate and have sex quite a bit. It's mainly in my bed though as I fall asleep so quickly.

Charlotte, 24, teacher, married 1 year

Our biggest problem is where, not if. I might be exaggerating a bit, but we are getting a bit more adventurous and it's become a bit of a game recently. I like sneaking in to her bed in the mornings and waking her with a cuddle, more often than not we end up having sex. But, we have started to look differently at various locations around the house. I can honestly say that it's been an unexpected bonus and I'm loving the fact that my wife is acting like we were when we started dating. I'm not sure how long this will last, but at this stage, I can't imagine not having sex with my wife – it would have to be that there was something really wrong between us, not because of our situation with beds.

Mike, 52, landscape gardener, married 23 years

> *Our marriage is not built on our sex life. There's so much more to us and who we are as a couple. There's still all the intimacy we want and need. Prior to recent illness we still had a very active sex life and separate beds have had nothing to do at all with a reduction in how often we have sex.*
> **John and Margaret, 58 and 50, married 30 years**

I hope these stories go some way to dispelling any myths or mistruths that sleeping separately means the end of the intimate side of a couple's relationship. Basically, if you are sleeping apart and not having sex it's because you have decided not to – not because you are victims of circumstance. In most instances, factors other than where you lay your head at night are far more likely to relegate your sex life to the bottom of the list of 'things I do with my partner'. Honestly, there are just as many couples sharing beds who rarely talk, kiss or cuddle and have a terrible or non-existent sex life.

We have to share a bed? Are you serious?

For waders and divers, another plan to be made is what to do if you both have to sleep in the same bed for one or more nights. This comes in to play if you visit friends or relatives and need to stay over, or the friends and relatives come to your place and need one of your rooms, or you go on holidays.

On a personal note, at all times Fraser and I try to arrange two rooms wherever we find ourselves sleeping at night. We are fortunate that both our parent's houses can accommodate our needs, but it's not always the case for staying with friends or when we go on holidays. We have accepted that our holidays can sometimes cost a little more if we want a two-bedroom unit. The argument then is who gets the bigger room – we take it in turns; very civil. However, when we stay in capital cities and want to be central, two rooms is an expense we can't stretch to. This is also an issue when we travel overseas. The main solution is for me to wear earplugs. However, as I've said, three nights is about my limit. There have been times where I have slept on couches if the accommodation permits, and I never underestimate the power of a few glasses of wine. We are quite active during the day on holidays and that certainly helps to wear me out. Sometimes though, I just don't get enough sleep, but I can live with that for a night or two, here and there.

Most couples interviewed used similar tactics. A common solution for families is that children (who seem to be able to sleep through just about anything) are split across two rooms, allowing the adults to split themselves across the rooms as well. Often noted is the ability to have an afternoon nap while on holidays, or recognition that not being at work means the need for an alert mind is not as imperative. However, there are solutions that are far more creative (although for some separate sleepers, holidays will never be what they once were).

> *I have sleeping tablets, specifically for the times when we have to share a bed on holidays. I use them for no other purpose except getting some sleep when I have to share a bed with my husband. Love him to death, by the way.*
>
> **Lulu, 42, legal professional, married 6 years**

> *On holidays, we try to split the sleeping across two rooms with one of the kids in a bed with each of us. If separate rooms are not an option then I bring ear plugs and industrial ear defenders from his workshop—the kind that someone uses when they are jackhammering. It probably seems hard to understand how I can sleep in them, but I position the pillow so that I can. I tested it with my snoring parents and it worked beautifully. Recently on a camping trip he knew he would keep everyone up in the cabin we had rented, so he slept outside in a tent.*
>
> **Suzette, 40, administrative assistant, married 17 years**

Holidays – I dread them! Why? If I want to sleep I have to wear ear plugs. Why should I have to do that? I have three children and I want to be able to hear if they need me. We recently went to Noosa for a night and thought we could surely spend one night in a bed together. Turns out – no, we can't. At about 3 am I'd had enough of the snoring (which of course he denied) so we had an argument and he ended up sleeping on the couch under one of my shirts.

Penny, 40, mother, married 14 years

Maintaining the plan

Once you have negotiated, refined and implemented the plan then you can sit back and relax – not. As social ecologist Peter Drucker says, 'Plans are only good intentions unless they immediately degenerate into hard work.' Many aspects of your relationship change as years pass and circumstances change. Relationships are not static; they constantly evolve so don't become complacent.

When you have a plan in place, whether it's version 1, 2, 2a or version 24, make the time to regularly check-in with your partner to monitor how successfully the new arrangements are working for both of you. You may have a wide grin on your face and look years younger because of nights of uninterrupted sleep, but also take a genuine interest in how they are feeling about the new regime.

Revisiting the key reasons of why you wanted to sleep separately and letting your partner know how it's working is an important part of the whole process – kind of like making sure your golf swing goes all the way round to the back of your body and doesn't stop half way just because you've hit the ball. Talking to your partner about any concerns that have developed, or indeed finding out if there are any positives they have discovered, will help to ensure the decisions made are sensible and potentially long-lasting.

Dr Timothy Sharp recommends that 'With any planning or goal setting one of the most important things to do is constantly review what has been agreed. Making the plan is not the end of it – a couple should regularly reconvene and review the plan. If there are warning signs or indications that it isn't working then they need to constantly evaluate, review and make changes so that it is working.'

> *When we finally decided to sleep apart, the first arrangement was Sunday–Thursday, so I could be rested for work. But after the first five to six months, I was beginning to dread Fridays because that was the night I would have to share with him. As much as I knew he would be upset, I just had to tell him that I couldn't do it. I had become used to having uninterrupted sleep so I figured why should I be exhausted on the weekends – that was my time to relax and do stuff, not spend Saturday and Sunday afternoons asleep to catch up. Loving someone does mean accepting them. I think my boyfriend has certainly had to learn that.*
> **Justine, 32, town planner**

Prioritising communication about your sleeping arrangements will ensure that you keep connected with your partner through a combined monitoring of the situation and sharing of how the change has affected you both. Keeping the communication flowing will also allow you to do any necessary tweaking of the arrangements. This is likely be new territory for both of you, and there is a strong chance you may not get it totally right to begin with, so you need to keep your minds and mouths open to work out the finer details and leave you both confident in your choices.

This tweaking might involve reminding your partner that they need to pop in and share a cuddle with you before you go to sleep, or you both agreed that for half an hour every night, you will turn the television off and just chat. Some fine-tuning of agreed behaviours might also be needed. For example, 'I know we said we would try and have a cuddle every night, but with all our activities during the week, meeting this commitment isn't working. If we can promise to do it on the weekends, is that going to be okay?'

Once you are sleeping according to the new rules, make sure that any boundaries and behaviours that were part of the deal are honoured by both of you. They can always be re-negotiated if they are not working but if you let them slip, you'll never really know if they were the right boundaries in the first place.

For example, the ritual of my morning kiss from my husband. The reason I wanted (and still do) a kiss in the morning was because I didn't want Fraser to get up and go to work without me being aware that he had left the house. My boundary there was about not missing out on the daily connections of life. There were a couple of times early in the arrangements that he said he didn't want to wake me to give me the kiss, but for me the kiss is more important than being woken – so he kisses me every morning. By way of a confessional – there have been maybe two or three times when we have been mid-fight and he hasn't kissed me because he is angry with me. From my perspective, the good thing about this is that it really alerts me to the seriousness of the argument – so it's kind of a bonus. Everyone's boundaries will be different in negotiating how to make separate sleeping work.

If you don't talk to your partner about how the plans are working, necessary changes might not happen and great successes may go uncelebrated; that would be a shame. Maybe you could arrange a conversation of this type with when you are having a cuddle on the couch, or one of you is visiting the other's room for some time together before you go to sleep?

> *There are times when we don't actually see or talk to each other for a few days because of my shifts and the fact that I'm downstairs and he's upstairs and we probably only eat together once a week. But John knows every move I make, my rosters, where I am, and I know where he is and what's happening in his life. Also, no major family decision would ever be made without a discussion between us taking place. This might mean that John comes to work to see me, we make the time for a phone call, or he comes early to catch me as none of these decisions are made independently. We respect each other too much.*
> **Margaret, 50, retail manager, married 30 years**

The bonus round

While there is a risk that the relationship might wobble a little when you move to separate rooms, there is also an equal possibility that one or both of you will find unexpected benefits when you experience single slumbering. All couples speak of the joy of having more sleep, but there's more to a bedroom than the sleeping.

> *I wake up earlier than Penny so I have found that what I really enjoy is the whole thing of making a coffee, taking it back to bed where I read a magazine or surf the web. That to me is the one thing I like and that I would really miss if I had to share a bed again. Sometimes I do it for about two hours while everyone else is asleep. I'm in bed, I'm warm and snug and I really enjoy it.*
> **Doug, 43, IT project manager, married 14 years**

> *Since I have the top floor of the house to myself now, I can have my bookcase in the lounge room with all my books in it, and*

all the sauce bottles and paper work for the business out in the kitchen. I always had to put those away. It's my den and it's become important to me.

John, 58, building contractor, married 30 years

Having never thought I would sleep in a separate room to my wife, I am surprised by how well it works for both of us. One thing I love is if I wake up at 3 am, I just reach over, get my iPad. It's great.

Richard, 46, sports professional, married 21 years

My room is so tidy now, and I have decorated the room in a more 'girly' way – I wasn't allowed to before. I feel like I was trapped for so long, it's like owning something for the first time, owning my own space – this is mine. I can decorate it how I want, be in it how I want. No water bottles, no watches, no eating in bed, no chocolate. I have flowers next to the bed and some crystals and all new sheets and pillows. I find the experience liberating.

Anne, 44, senior manager, married 20 years

Since Sophie moved to the other room, I actually don't mind. I had always thought we would be sleeping together because it's the traditional thing to do, but this arrangement is actually working well for us both. I sleep when I sleep, I can get up and get a drink of water, go to the toilet ... I can do what I want. I'm probably sleeping a fair bit better because it's less disturbed sleep. I'm passively enjoying it. I get up at strange hours so it's convenient for me. I can get up early and then come back to bed again and it doesn't disturb either of us. It's great.

Anthony, 62, education professional, married 25 years

What happens when the plan isn't working?

As Thomas Edison said: 'I have not failed. I've just found 10,000 ways that won't work.' This chapter focuses unashamedly on solutions and success. However, we all know that plans can fail. In your path to separate sleeping nirvana you are likely to encounter some bumps along the way. Some people might find mountains, and some may never solve their sleeping issues. Not every story has a happy ending. If you aren't finding your happy ending, you may need to look further than this book, as the issues are possibly bigger than where you lay your head at night. Sometimes just speaking to your GP is a good place to start.

When you are planning though, include some thinking and talking about what might go wrong. Any good contract lawyer would support me in this advice. If you can foresee and prepare for pitfalls, the disappointment and frustration when they happen will be lessened.

The foreseen problems will range in scale, which will have an impact on how easily they can be solved. For example, smaller issues might arise, such as:

- When one of you wants to come into the other's bed but the other doesn't want them in there.
- When neither of you wants to volunteer to move to the spare room.
- If neither of you wants give up your room when you have so many guests that a surrender of one of your beds is required.
- If one of you feels they got a raw deal by not having access to cupboards or ensuite.
- If the person in the main room feels as though they are still being disturbed by the other coming in to the room to get clothes, have a shower etc.

While smaller issues can have simple solutions, there may be some problems that are harder to resolve or situations where one of you is happy with the changes but the other one isn't. How would you deal with the situation when one of you:

- doesn't like sleeping apart
- feels that you are growing apart
- is unhappy about changes to your sex life and the romance and physical aspects of the relationship
- feels that the arrangements agreed upon aren't working anymore
- can't deal with questions about the new arrangements?

These tough problems may not have quick, easy resolutions. They may require some external advice, but continuing to support, communicate and be open and honest with each other will certainly help as you work your way through these issues.

PAUSE FOR THOUGHT...

☾ Is your relationship in a place and space to be making plans to sleep separately?

☾ Does where you live offer some options to accommodate sleeping separately?

☾ How well do you and your partner plan for upcoming events? And more importantly, how well do you cope and deal with each other, and the situation, if a plan doesn't work?

☾ Do you know already if you are heading for the paddling or wading pool, or are you limbering up for an elegant dive into the deep end? And does your partner know about your plans? If not, how is he going to find out?

☾ How do you and your partner define intimacy? Is this something you can talk to them about if you were to sleep separately?

☾ Are you in a position to accommodate all the logistics of the plans you are making for your changed sleeping arrangements?

☾ Is there a trusted friend or family member that could help you come up with some creative suggestions to your particular sleep plan if you are stuck when thinking of solutions? How could you approach this person if you needed to?

7

What will the neighbours think?

'It is grossly selfish to require of one's neighbour that he should think in the same way, and hold the same opinions. Why should he? If he can think, he will probably think differently. If he cannot think, it is monstrous to require thought of any kind.' – Oscar Wilde

Our Sleeping Separately Checklist

1. Recognise and understand the need for sleep ☑
2. Have well-prepared discussion with partner ☑
3. Reach consensus on what needs to change ☑
4. Plan changes.... with partner (including contingencies) ☑
5. Tell others about our decision... ❓

When you have made the decision to sleep separately there will come a time when you may want to tell people what's happened, or you are put in a position where the new arrangements are uncovered and you either choose to spill the beans about who is sleeping in which bed at your house, or are left in a situation where you have little choice but to do so. As with many other aspects of sleeping separately the sharing experience will be different for everyone. For some, telling others of your decision may cause as much disruption to your life as swatting away a fly, but for others letting people know of the new arrangements is more difficult than making the decision itself. Why? It's all tangled up in our version of what makes a successful life and wanting other people to think we're successful too.

A fundamental feature of humans is we want to be liked. Some of us are satisfied knowing there is just one person in the world who enjoys our company, whereas others require an entourage to pander them 24/7. Maslow's ubiquitous triangle of needs has been telling us for decades that once we have all the basics in place (of which sleep is found on the foundation layer I might add), then we work to meet a range of other needs further up the pyramid. At the pointy end of the triangle are self-esteem, confidence, and respect from others, which are all gained through positive interactions with people that like us.

Seeking approval from others helps us meet Maslow's higher order needs by making us feel good about ourselves, proud of our achievements, relevant to others' lives and valued by the people we care about – and there's no harm in admitting that. To have our needs met we tend to behave in ways that we hope will continue to make us an attractive proposition. We work hard for our boss, we follow our parents' rules, we give our friends presents for their birthdays and engage in all sorts of social behaviours to oil the wheels of happy relationships and keep the ones we're out to impress coming back for more.

On a very basic level we form two types of relationships in our lives. There are the ones over which we have little or no control – family, co-workers, neighbours. Then there are the ones we manage ourselves – friends and intimate partners. While I don't intend to go into the complexities of the interpersonal dynamics of all types of relationships, it is sufficient to say that when we seek approval (in whatever form) from any person, our behaviour is influenced to obtain that approval. What we say and do, how we act, our opinions shared and unspoken and our appearance, whether in clothes or deeds, are open to influence when we want someone to tell us that we are okay. It's the reason we all have photos of ourselves sporting questionable fashion trends from the past which make us cringe with embarrassment when they appear in a photo slide show at our fortieth birthday party.

Some argue that being validated through others' approval is one of the strongest motivating forces known to man. However, on a day-to-day basis just knowing that there are people who like you, and seek you out for a chat or a hug, can provide you with the necessary emotional and physical nourishment needed to encourage you to hop out of bed each morning.

Social approval is just as important. Psychologists describe social approval as a need, not a desire, and a psychological reality for healthy self-esteem. As social beings, our need to belong to a group starts young and stays forever. Again, it's an issue that's danced around many wise brains and filled many university libraries, so not one I'm going to delve into too deeply here. But it does have an influence on the topic of this book. As has been noted, sleeping is a social behaviour that attracts social scrutiny. As a result, people around us feel that they can comment on our sleeping practices and therefore give us the 'stamp of approval, or the sigh of dismay', depending on what your bedroom behaviours are and what they think of them.

> *Our friends were interested to see that we had separate rooms and thought 'Well, this marriage is on its way out'.*
> **Von, 72, married 55 years**

A contributing factor to how much value you place on the approval of others is their relative importance in your life. The more important people are to you, the more value you place on the relationship and the greater their approval matters, or, better put, the more their disapproval matters.

So when you and your partner are with other people and say, 'Hey, X and I have decided to move into separate rooms', how will the people in your life react? Will their reaction influence your behaviour and how you feel about the decision you've made?

Oh the stigma of it all!

Let's get right down to it! The most common reason that separate sleeping is maligned is the stigma that says if you're sleeping separately, your relationship is in trouble – people speculate about the cause, from issues with your sex life to the end of the relationship. And there's no real surprise in that conclusion. A common response when two people engage in conflict is to avoid each other, so the judgement does have a sound anthropological basis.

> *An aunt who is 15 years older than me passed a comment on my husband and I sleeping in separate rooms – 'If we slept in separate beds that would be the end of our relationship'. I did worry about what she had said for a while, but I couldn't draw a comparison to my relationship and our situation. My uncle doesn't snore, which is a big difference.*
> **Leanne, 41, HR executive, married 15 years**

However, as with all generalisations we are subjected to and subject others to, there are exceptions. So why can't we make the decision to sleep separately, then say to all those judgers and detractors, 'Don't worry, everything's okay' and just get on with it?

Well, lots of people do, and their friends and family are convinced over time that everything is indeed okay and they aren't facing the support tasks that come along with the end of an intimate relationship. This was certainly my situation, and nine years on, I think I've convinced everyone that Fraser and I are okay, which is a relief.

However, the social groupings some people find themselves in may not accept a simple statement of 'everything's okay'. Stop and think about some really strong opinions you have. What are they? For me, I am quite firm in the belief that every person has the right to a good night's sleep, as evidenced by what you are reading.

Most people have an opinion about what constitutes a 'good marriage' or a 'good relationship'. The notion of pairing with another in a committed relationship brings the expectation that you will spend a lot of time together, and be each other's social partner of choice, operating as a unit in life. It's not an unrealistic model given the cultural and social messages in the media and society. When this typical model is not adhered to, eyebrows begin to rise and murmurs of 'What's wrong?' start.

> *Some people I tell find it so confronting. When people hear we have separate rooms, immediately you see their faces drop and think 'Oh, there's something wrong with the marriage, why haven't you told me?' Women have taken me aside and asked if everything is okay. I didn't even think it would be an issue for other people, but I would see the shock on their faces.*
> **Penny, 40, mother of 3, married 10 years**

> *I don't know if I would tell anyone because I wouldn't want them to think there was something wrong with us. I don't want them to jump to the wrong conclusions – that there is something wrong, because there isn't.*
> **Sophie, 60, retired, married 25 years**

> *Recently I mentioned to a friend that my husband and I sleep separately. 'Oh, are you okay?' was her immediate reaction. I said we were fine and mentioned we were building another*

bedroom and she totally assumed that we were having marital problems. I told her that there were absolutely no problems and that it was more about the fact that I don't want to kill my husband because I am sleep deprived.
Suzette, 40, administrative assistant, married 17 years

I don't promote or advertise it at all as people will think there are cracks and vulnerabilities in the relationship – it's nobody else's business and I don't want people to judge us on that. If it comes up, it's not a secret, but I find it very personal.
Amelia, 41, mother of two, married 12 years

I don't necessarily care if people know. I don't go out of my way to tell people, but don't deny it. I don't have a problem talking about it. I think people who react negatively to it are very old fashioned. It's nothing to be ashamed of at all – it's just practical. When my parents did it, it just made sense.
Maree and John, 30 and 33, health professionals, married 3 years

I'm very open about our situation so get some interesting reactions. People say 'It's not a real marriage', but I tell them 'Different strokes for different folks and it's what works for us'.
Caroline, 30, photographer, married 7 years

A 2007 article from the *New York Times* considered the point of view of builders and architects who were engaged by people building and renovating to accommodate their separate sleeping needs. Even these people recognised the issues faced by people when it came to sharing their decision.

> *Many architects and designers say their clients believe there is still a stigma to sleeping separately. Some developers say it is a delicate issue and call the other bedroom a 'flex suite' for when the in-laws visit or the children come home from college. Charles Brandt, an interior designer in St. Louis said, 'The builder*

> knows, the architect knows, the cabinet maker knows, but it's not something they like to advertise because right away people will think something is wrong with the marriage'.

So many images in Western culture depict a good relationship by showing a happy couple jumping into a bed together every night. So it's really no surprise that so many people take their cues of what to do to be a good couple from these images and are challenged by a different model. When faced with a different way of doing life well, some people become fearful. The unknown is a scary place and some of us don't want our happy, successful life model tested by others. Because what if my model fails? Better the devil you know than the devil you don't!

For some, the sting of the stigma is closer to home and comes from themselves. Messages throughout their lives have told them that a couple should sleep together, and they may have judged others in the past on unconventional decisions that didn't fit with their own model. So when faced with the situation where they are the ones not living up to their own ideals of a good relationship, the internal conflict can send them into shame and guilt, making sure that any sleeping arrangements outside the norm remain secret.

> *I would fret about it and think that I was a bad wife because the only time my parents ever slept apart was when they were having a fight and my mother locked my father out of the room. I have been brought up to believe that in a family, parents do everything together, they sleep together, they get up and make the bed together – that's what a good couple do. I don't think I will ever tell my parents that I am sleeping apart from my husband. I have only told one person at work that my husband and I have moved to separate rooms. There's a stigma that says there's something wrong that we aren't sleeping together and*

> *I don't think I'll ever be comfortable about being in separate rooms. However, I do find the experience liberating.*
> **Anne, 44, senior manager, married 20 years**

Realistically, the best way to chip away at the stigma that your relationship is in its death throes because you aren't sleeping in the same bed is with ongoing successful separate sleeping. The longer you sleep apart and stay together, the quieter the naysayers become. (And maybe give them a copy of this book)

What about my BFFs?

When we are young our friendship groups happen to us, not by us. Friends appear in our life because of who we sit next to in class, who our mum makes friends with at the school gate or tuckshop and who we live next door to. As we grow older, friendships are made more independently, through shared values, social norms and social behaviours.

There is a wealth of psychology behind why we make friends with one person rather than another – but it's basically because they are like us and they get us. They get our sense of humour, our social decisions and they like the things we like. Often there are characteristics we see in our friends that we would like for ourselves and that also attract us to them. Essentially, you share a certain amount of social assets with this person, so you hang out. Friends validate each other. That's why you seek them out over others, because you are always approving of each other and have a lot of fun together.

Sometimes we make friends for aspirational reasons. We may seek out people in a different demographic to ourselves because they represent the type of person we want to be, or we are presented with an opportunity to mix with a group of people who are different to us, and all of a sudden we have a different set of norms to learn about and demonstrate if we want to remain in the gang. These types of friendships may not have the foundations that allow for a level of honesty that you might have with other friends, but there is something in the social pairing you want, and one of those things is their approval.

Friends have their opinions too, and sometimes we find ourselves on the outer edge of a group because we aren't modelling the requisite behaviour to belong. We aren't wearing the right brand of clothes, being seen at the right restaurants or parties, drinking at the right bars or hotels, supporting the right football code (or even knowing what codes there are and that we are supposed to support a team) – or we aren't sleeping in the same bed as our partner.

I have a friend who found herself in a mother's group arranged through her local baby clinic after the birth of her first child. These were not people she would necessarily choose to be her friends. She told me she felt like a terrible mother because her child, four to five months old at that point, wasn't sleeping through the night when all the other babies in her mother's group were. Now, I'm not a mother myself, but I have many friends who are, so I knew that when their children were four to five months old, they didn't generally sleep through the night. When I told her this, she conceded that she had thought the mothers who were saying this might not have been completely honest. She felt they were trying to give the impression that their child was perfect, ergo they were a good mum. The sad thing was she started to lie about her child's sleep so she too could receive the praise and approval of the other mothers and be included in the conversations about how good it was to be getting a full night's sleep and how much happier her baby was the next day. Her need for approval from these mothers was such that she not only lied about the reality of her situation, but she felt she was a failure because she couldn't live up to their unrealistic expectations. My heart went out to her as she cried about the situation. Not only was she giving herself a really bad time, she was absolutely exhausted because her baby kept her awake most nights.

There are people who like to present a façade of blissful happiness in their domestic life. For some it's a very shiny badge of honour. What is a blissful domestic life though? There's the one often portrayed in the media of mum and dad being terribly good at whatever domestic arrangement works for them – both working or mum at home with dad as the breadwinner – the kids are happy and healthy, everyone gets on with each other, a fluffy dog plays enthusiastically in the back yard and everyone has an untroubled life. (Just to confirm – mum and dad do sleep in the same bed every night, very happily, with lots of pillows and a great matching doona and sheet set and coordinated, stylish nightwear.)

If this is your family and you are happy, then great! There is nothing wrong with this story, but it's just not everyone's story and there would be a lot of people who don't want that story either. What's blissful to one is not blissful to another and neither state of bliss is better than the other. The different definitions of blissful are what enables frameworks for judgement and disapproval. If you have friends, who either through actions or words, make it very clear they would never sleep separately to their partner, then it might be difficult to come clean that you do – if you fear that they will disapprove of your decision. It's even tougher if you think that their disapproval might lead them to judge you negatively and not seek out your friendship anymore.

> *We don't tell a lot of people that we sleep in separate rooms. We had to put a system in place because sleeping together wasn't working. My room still looks like a spare room anyway, so no-one would notice the difference.*
>
> **May, 66, retired, married 40 years**

> *I've told my two best friends and that's it. I don't need to be judged and I know I have friends who will do that. When I'm with friends and they are joking and laughing about their husbands snoring and keeping them awake at night I join in. I have years of experience to keep telling stories. What would happen if they found out? I'll cross that bridge when I come to it, but I do think about that happening from time to time.*
>
> **Maddie, 35, health professional, married 6 years**

We don't like to think of ourselves as failures. And keeping friendships is a task at which we can fail. Sometimes our friends, their reactions to what we do and their opinions about us act as a social mirror. So when you normalise your behaviour against people you consider your friends, but who have a different normal to you, you may not feel comfortable looking in that mirror. When it comes to sharing that you can't sleep with your partner any more, you need to decide if sharing the information and risking disapproval is the right thing for you, or if you prefer to keep that type of information to yourself. Dr Timothy Sharp says that in the majority of circumstances, most people outside a relationship don't know the ins and outs of how it works and they don't need to. As in many other areas of your life, how important is it what other people think of you? It's a balancing act but what's important to you and your partner should be the main priority to focus on.

> *My husband was out with his mates and telling them a story about how our son prefers my pink sheets to his blue sheets. When they found out the sheets were different colours because we have separate rooms they thought it was the weirdest thing ever and couldn't believe that we sleep in separate beds. In fact, lots of our friends question it or are really shocked and surprised by it. They think it's the strangest thing they have ever heard.*
>
> **Charlotte, 24, teacher, married 1 year**

> *Like any man, I of course like the idea of going to bed next to and waking up next to my wife every day. This is what I have always equated to normal. It makes me sad when I wake up in the morning and she is gone. It makes me frustrated when she wakes me up in the night and asks me to leave. I understand that sleeping together many nights is just near on impossible for her with my restlessness and snoring and she reaches a breaking point. I understand; but it still upsets me. We've had many conversations together about how we need to create a new kind of 'normal' that works for us. But I have to be honest; I would definitely feel embarrassed telling my mates that my wife and I don't share a bed most nights. It's the ridicule and them asking 'What's wrong with you mate?' that is still hard to face.*
>
> **Harold, 33, business development manager, married 1 year**

Who you do and don't tell is an individual decision. You will know which of your friends will cope and which ones will feel challenged. Consider however, that there may be friends who although presenting a façade of happy home with perfectly sleeping babies and super happy husbands snoozing the nights away next to them, may be thrilled to hear there are options available for them to get a good night's sleep. They might be grateful that someone has the courage to be honest about the issue and follow your lead.

There may also be people who are grateful to have the opportunity to discuss the idea of separate sleeping with you. It gives them the opportunity to find out how it can work and how it might affect a relationship, positively or otherwise.

> *Even though we have had problems sharing a bed for a while now, I really hadn't thought about moving to separate rooms until I spoke to a friend and found out he was doing it. I guess I just didn't think it was an option. I started telling my wife about what my friend did and after a few conversations we thought*

I should move to the spare room downstairs. I love it, my wife loves it. It's great. We've got a friend coming to stay for a few weeks soon and I have to move back to the main room for that time. I'm not looking forward to having to give up my room.

Richard, 46, sports professional, married 21 years

I have had lots of interesting things said to me as I am very open about it. Some people are shocked, some people have said they wished they had separate rooms and others have then gone out and done the same thing.

Melissa, 47, executive, married 27 years

Often when I'm with friends we will get on to the topic of snoring and it often leads to 'Where do you sleep at night'. Sometimes the question comes up 'Does your wife put up with it?' Some say 'Yes', and some say 'No, I have to sleep in another room.' It's as simple as that. We're all in the same boat. I feel good to know there are others in the same situation as me. None of my friends say they are in another room for any other reason so I don't know of any other. We talk seriously about it. If there are other people around it can be a bit light-hearted, but one-on-one the conversations can get serious. Some wished that they didn't have to be out of their own rooms, some miss their wives. No-one's embarrassed; they are more concerned about whether it's impacted on their intimacy. In some cases it has and they want to talk about it. What they are looking for is – it is the same for you? Is everything alright? And they are not as intimate – but for them, there are probably other factors that impact on the fact their intimacy is not as they want it. It's definitely more than just sleeping in separate rooms. I've probably spoken to about three close friends about it and we do agree that we don't like keeping our wives awake, but don't have issues with sex.

Matt, 47, senior manager, married 20 years

Those close to you may not be the only people with whom you choose to share your separate sleeping news. While most people don't go out of their way to constantly announce their night-time domestic arrangements, there may be times where the topic is raised, or an opening for a discussion on the issue presents itself and before you know it, you're sharing your personal story with someone you've just met. As a veteran of this practice, I have some advice on the array of responses that you might be presented with as well as how to deal with them if you do choose the virtuous path of truth as a separate sleeper.

You do what?

While I never start a conversation with, 'Hi, I'm Jenny and I sleep in a separate room to my husband,' I certainly don't shy away from talking about this aspect of my life. Often in conversation I will mention 'my husband's bedroom' or 'my bedroom', or the context of the conversation is such that the topic is appropriate to broach. Having a particular interest in alternative sleeping arrangements, I enjoy hearing other people's view on the practice. I also enjoy hearing their stories as separate sleepers or dedicated co-sleepers themselves. I am interested in hearing anecdotes about how the range of sleeping misdemeanours is managed by couples. There is also a cheeky side of me that enjoys challenging social norms, so I bring an enthusiastic interest to the debate of 'one bed or two'.

These are the most common responses I have encountered. You may recognise some of these – and be able to add some more types to the list.

The Head Tilter

As this person listens to you explain that you sleep separately to your partner, their head starts to tilt – not too much, to either the left or the right. You are left thinking – is there something wrong with your neck? While there may indeed be a spine-related injury they're dealing with, the Centre for Non-verbal Studies says that a head tilt can be used to show friendliness or be one of several self-protective gestures.

Potentially, these people think your relationship is in such dire straits that you need more friends. Or maybe they are thinking, 'I wonder if my partner wants to sleep separately from me?' So the head is tilted as a pre-emptive pose that will enable them to spring into action in case this is a reality. I am conjecturing, of course.

Over time I have attempted to drill down and uncover the Tilter's motivation, but I have been unable to elicit responses from people that fit with either of the above two explanations of this non-verbal behaviour. To date, no-one has invited me to the movies or a picnic, or to hang out with them, and no-one has fled in terror, fearful that I would convince their partner to join the cause. I guess that's the thing about non-verbal cues – often the words that accompany the non-verbals are at odds with the gesture so these people can be confusing. Needless to say, you have the Tilter thinking about something or they wouldn't have struck such a pose.

There is a tilt that I call the 'pity tilt' – you can see it in their eyes. Often the Tilter tries to encourage an admission from you that there must be just a little something wrong with the relationship for you to take such drastic steps. I have had a couple of Tilters encourage me to admit to them that there is something wrong in my marriage. 'It's okay, you can tell me' has been offered as a safe haven for my confession. 'Don't you miss the cuddles all night?' they coo. 'Don't you want to snuggle next to your husband, fall asleep and wake up next to him in the morning?' The answers to these questions are 'yes' and 'yes', hastily followed by 'but what is more important to us is getting enough sleep to function, etc'.

How to respond to a Tilter: What I would love to do is reach over to the Tilter and straighten their head for them, but there are all sorts of issues such as social boundaries and good manners I would break if I did that. We know you can't change opinions in one conversation, so my response to them (and it's going to be a repeated suggestion in the next couple of pages) is to assure the Tilter that all is well in your relationship, this is the solution that works well for you and your partner, and as individuals, we have the ability to make decisions that work best for us. You might also offer the Tilter some more information about sleeping separately – possibly throw in a few statistics – so they have a greater understanding of people who are in a happy relationship, but just can't sleep in the same bed at night. It's just logic, not the end of the world.

The Seat Shifter

Seat Shifters do not want to hear about your separate sleeping. There is something about the practice that unnerves them so that they start moving around in their seat and employ every non-verbal tactic available to let you know you have strayed into taboo territory with them. Most commonly, they will move from an open body position to a cross-legged one that has the leg closest to you crossed away from you. They will angle their body away from you as well. This can be uncomfortable if you are in a small group.

Next comes the gentle, polite, winding down of the conversation. They will stop talking as much as they were, and move to 'mmms' and nods as you continue to try to engage them in the conversation they appeared to be quite happy having about three minutes ago.

Being a mostly polite girl, I respect these cues and finish the topic as seamlessly as I can, letting the Seat Shifter return to a happy space by moving the conversation on to the weather or a recent sporting event.

An educated guess tells me that this topic is off limits for them. Not wanting to exacerbate their uncomfortableness I have never pursued Seat Shifters to find out why they respond so. Whether it touches on a boundary of what constitutes their version of a good relationship, or crosses the line of what's appropriate to talk about in polite company, or is something they do but don't want to disclose ... who knows?

How to respond to a Seat Shifter: I really do think the best thing to do is be as polite as you can and gently move away from the topic. If the Seat Shifter wants to talk about it again, they will – that has happened once to me. Everyone's level of social comfort around personal topics is different, and it is important to respect that. Depending on where you are in the conversation, it could be worthwhile to drop in that your relationship is okay. This would help Seat Shifters to feel that they could get back to you if there was something they wanted to know or talk about further with you.

The Frowner

The Frowner is similar to the Tilter but has a more judgemental edge. Whereas the Tilter might be overcome with pity and want to take you home and cuddle you all night in bed, the Frowner is usually communicating that 'couples don't sleep separately'. A frown unarguably says disapproval, so the Frowner is sharing their disapproval and displeasure at what you are telling them. They don't feel uncomfortable; they feel self-righteous and confident that their opinion on the practice is the right one, and guess what? You have it all wrong.

The Frowner is as confident about why you shouldn't sleep separately as you are about why you should, so this one could be a battle of wills if you want to engage them. I like engaging Frowners as all views and thoughts about couples sleeping together intrigue me. If you are feeling a bit provocative and up for a rowdy and robust discussion, the Frowner is a great sparring partner.

Be careful though, the Frowner might be a version of the Seat Shifter and their disapproval is actually about raising such a personal topic when you don't know them all that well. You may have caught them off guard and while their level of discomfort is not as pronounced as the Seat Shifter's, the frown might be enough of a cue for you to look outside and see what the clouds are up to.

How to respond to the Frowner: First, if you think the Frowner is disapproving of the practice of separate sleeping, you might want to gird your loins and take them on in a feisty debate, or depending on the context, back down and pull out that trusty weather conversation. Second, if the frown emanates because of the personal nature of the topic, or the time and place of the conversation, changing to an innocuous topic will allay their concern and hopefully have them using their best smiling muscles within seconds.

The Secret Sharer

The Secret Sharer is one of my personal favourites. They often listen intently to the explanation of your sleeping arrangements because they too are separate sleepers but don't tell anyone. They question your motivations, how you made it happen, how your relationship is going now, but what they most want to know is how you go about telling other people. Do you tell other people? What do you say? What do the other people say?

Are you embarrassed? What do your parents think? What do your friends think? What do the pets think? Where do the pets sleep? What do the kids think? Have you told your workmates? What did they say? How many people do you tell? Why? Depending on their enthusiasm, it can be hard to get a word in.

Because Secret Sharers are separate sleepers themselves – some in the wading pool, some in the deep end – they want to know how you manage the fact that other people know about your separate sleeping. They want to know this because they don't tell anyone about their separate sleeping. Whether they are looking for a roadmap for how to tell others, or they want to vicariously revel in the social freedom you enjoy, they just can't get enough of your war stories of disclosure.

The Secret Sharer will often take the opportunity to disclose to you that they too sleep separately. This will only happen in a one-on-one situation. If you start your story in a group of people, the Secret Sharer will wait until they can capture you alone to quietly say, 'My partner and I sleep separately too'. What you then have is a sharing of details and the opportunity to make someone's day and normalise their life. I always feel honoured when a Secret Sharer confides in me, but I must admit I do tend to keep them cornered too, to drill down into why they reluctant to share their situation. Much like the Frowner, they have a story to tell, and I am always genuinely interested in hearing the story.

How to respond to the Secret Sharer: First and foremost – don't break their confidence. It's a privilege to have someone share such personal details with you and not one to be taken lightly. By explaining your thought processes about why it's okay to share your situation with others, you help the Secret Sharer see that there is a social acceptance of the practice that can be gained from assuring others that separate beds don't mean the end of the relationship. Without patronising the Secret Sharer, find a way to affirm their sharing. I have never taken on the role of a separate sleeping evangelist, so am not inclined to free them from their shackles of shame and personally, I don't think after hearing their confession, that introducing them to others as, 'This is Pete. He's a teacher and a father of three and hasn't slept in the same bed as his wife for the last five years' is the right thing to do. I advise affirming their choice and teaching him the 'separate sleeper secret sign' – just kidding. That hasn't been designed yet.

The I-want-to-hug-you

I-want-to-hug-you listens to your story with a look of immediate empathy and warmth. They may reach out and touch you on the arm, or put their hand to their mouth as they take little gasps at each revelation you share. When you have told enough of your story for them to realise how similar their story is to yours, they will disclose that they too are a separate sleeper. I-want-to-hug-you is more likely than the Secret Sharer to disclose there and then, irrespective of company, that they are in the club.

I-want-to-hug-you is just so glad to hear that there are others out there that share their situation and they wants to show you how much they appreciates the camaraderie by adding a physical element to the conversation – this is when the hug or the further arm touch might happen. You may actually be the first person that I-want-to-hug-you has come out to, so don't treat their sharing lightly. They are not as embarrassed about their choice as Secret Sharer, but being human, they appreciate the chance to normalise a behaviour they may previously have thought they were the only ones engaging in.

Similarly, I-want-to-hug-you might latch on to you and want to know more because they hadn't even thought that this option was available to them. In fact, if this is the case, they may cry when they hug you because a light in their otherwise darkened, sleep-deprived life has been turned on by your sharing. Depending on your own social boundaries, you have to decide how you manage a teary, but grateful stranger.

How to respond to I-want-to-hug-you: We all like to know we're not alone in the world, especially when we choose a path less travelled. We want to meet the other travellers on our narrow path. It's exciting when we do. Welcome I-want-to-hug-you with as much enthusiasm as you are comfortable displaying. The SSC (Separate Sleepers Club) has a membership equivalent to only 25 per cent of most Western cultures, so while an important group in society (because we're so well-rested and therefore highly functioning social contributors) we aren't the majority. I-want-to-hug-you might want to share the details of their story with you, so plan ahead for meeting this person and think about how much you want to share and hear.

The Overly-Interested Questioner

Overly-Interested Questioners wants to hear all the details about your separate sleeping arrangements for one of two reasons. Either they are thinking about doing it or their partner has been talking about doing it. Overly-Interested Questioners are on a fact-finding mission and you have presented yourself as a personal 'Separate Sleeping Wikipedia' page. They are not going to miss this chance to click every hyperlink in your brain. Once you identify the Overly-Interested Questioner it's your chance to speak proudly and confidently about your arrangements. These people are great to engage in conversation because you have something they want, so you are in the driver's seat.

You may want to take your time as you meticulously outline your separate sleeping arrangements and how it's been a life-changing experience for you, or choose a *Reader's Digest* version to give them a taste of what life could be like for them.

You may indeed choose to hand the driver's seat over to the Overly-Interested Questioner and let them probe your expert knowledge bank. Whatever method you choose, it might be a good idea to get comfortable.

How to respond to the Overly-Interested Questioner: Be ready with facts. Also be ready to answer a lot of questions that might plumb un-thought of depths in terms of detail. Consider asking them questions yourself to help them clarify their lines of enquiry. Be patient with Overly-Interested Questioners – they may be developing the questions on the run, so won't always be precise and methodical in their approach. And I warn you again, find a comfortable spot: you might be there for a while.

The That's-Interesting-Tell-Me-More

These people are simply interested in hearing your story, and your thoughts about separate sleeping. They don't judge, they just listen. That's-Interesting-Tell-Me-Mores may be separate sleepers or they may not. They are just folk who are keen to have a good chat about a sociological behaviour and hear what other people in the world are up to. No surprises, no twist in the tail.

How to respond to That's-Interesting-Tell–Me-More: Enjoy!

Doin' it for the kids

How you treat the task of telling your children about mum and dad's sleeping arrangements depends on the age of your children. If you have been sleeping separately since your children were youngsters then you may only have to explain the situation if they ask questions following a sleepover at a friend's place where 'My friend's parents do this really weird thing and sleep together'.

> *After taking questions from a friend about the stability of my relationship because my husband and I weren't sleeping in the same room she then asked, 'How do the kids feel about it?' I explained that it happened when my older one was five or six years old, so the kids don't know any different.*
> **Suzette, 40, administrative assistant, married 17 years**

> *Our kids think it's completely normal. They might think that sharing a room with a partner is abnormal.*
> **Melissa, 47, executive, married 27 years**

However, any explanation to young ones will probably be the same, no matter whether you are letting them know of an impending move to separate rooms or are giving them a rationale for your decision. This is another one of those situations where you will know what is best for you and your children, so you are in complete control in regards to the level of detail you share and the emotion you create in explaining the situation. Their age and understanding of the dynamics of a mummy/daddy relationship will obviously impact on these factors.

Much like the concern raised by adults, some children might look at mummy and daddy heading to a different room at night and wonder if it might be leading to different houses in the not too distant future – 'like it did for Billy and Belinda at school'. Obviously, the key information that children need is to know that mummy and daddy are okay. This is easily evidenced by ensuring there are lots of cuddles and kisses between you, and again, depending on their level of understanding, having a discussion with your children about the stability of a relationship not being affected by where you sleep at night.

> *I constructed a story of the King and Queen's chambers for our children. So when they come into my bed in the morning on the weekends they think it's fun to come into the Queen's bed.*

> *When the King then comes in too, they think it's even better. They see that mummy and daddy still love each other because we're all in mummy's bed together laughing. <u>Sometimes they go into Doug's bed too for a chat in the mornings</u>.*
> **Penny, 40, mother of 3, married 10 years**

At a minimum, don't leave children wondering why their mummy and daddy are different to their friends' mummies and daddies who sleep in the same bed each night. And discussing the issue also presents an opportunity to teach your children that not everyone is exactly the same and that relationships can be successful in many different ways.

Another situation you may find yourself facing is the inquisitiveness of friends of your children during sleepovers at your house. While it isn't up to you to educate other people's kids about the birds and bees, you don't want your children to feel uncomfortable if their friends question, what is to them a strange arrangement. Something as simple as 'We sleep in separate rooms because we keep each other awake' is all that is needed to allay concerns. You may also want to coach your children to provide a simple explanation to their friends if the need arises. You may also choose to say nothing unless questions are asked by children or their parents.

> *When our children had friends coming to stay over I would see them looking perplexed that their friend's mum and dad were going to separate rooms when they went to bed. I could see them trying to process 'so the mum's bedroom is upstairs and the dad's is downstairs'. I think my kids just explained that it was normal in our house and it didn't really seem to bother them.*
> **Brooke, 52, educational professional, married 30 years**

Be mindful of your own child's developmental stage, as we all remember the cringe-worthy things our parents said to our friends. It would be nice if you could avoid making your child a social pariah with an overly-detailed explanation of you and your partner's personal issues.

Be strong, stay strong and sleep well

Greek philosopher Heraclitus left us with the iconic quote that 'The only constant in life is change'. This is certainly the case with social behaviour. Humans don't stop evolving and how we socialise has always been and will always be an area of change and challenge. We have evolved from sleeping separately to snuggling in a small space together, but maybe that is not proving to be the solution for everyone anymore. Klösch notes that 'Separate bedrooms are becoming less of a taboo topic for couples. Separate sleeping arrangements are being chosen more and more often by pairs, and not just because of snoring... the double bed and sleeping together as a pair are products of cultural and historical processes, not biological necessity.' He goes on to say 'The days are gone when sharing a bed was seen as an indication of the health of the relationship ... separate beds and bedrooms can be a clear and visible sign of a lively and dynamic relationship.'

> *I think a marriage is whatever two people decide it is. It's what they decide what works for them. But a lot of people are worried about what the impression is that they give to others for fear of what will be said. I do feel that my husband is uncomfortable with it being an open topic, so I wouldn't raise it to prevent him feeling awkward.*
> **Kaye, 66, together 14 years**

> *We only tell people if it comes up. A lot of friends and all of our extended family know what we do and why we do it. I think our attitude and approach to the situation makes other people*

> *feel okay about what we are doing. <u>They see our relationship is okay, so we think that puts them at ease.</u> We sleep in separate rooms because it's convenient for us. That's what we tell people.*
>
> Richard and Catherine, 48 and 46, IT engineer and health professional, married 20 years

If you know that sleeping separately to your partner is the right choice for you and for your physical and mental health then be confident in that decision. There is no compulsion to share the decision or the details if you don't want to. But know that the decision is the right one for you and don't feel as though you have to justify it – publically or silently – because it's different to the norm.

If you are confident that the reason you and your partner sleeping separately is not to create a smokescreen for bigger issues in your relationship, then that needs to be evident when you talk about what you are doing. If you feel you are sleeping separately because there are bigger issues in your relationship then it's probably a good idea to get brave and deal with those issues.

Telling others is all in the delivery. Share it nervously and it will be received that way. Share it calmly and assuredly, and while you may not invoke immediate acceptance and approval from those who doubt or disapprove, you will at least begin the conversation with them from a better starting point. Many times words are ignored when they are overshadowed by the vibe we pick up from the person who is telling us something. How you feel about your separate sleeping will influence your 'vibe', so think about your non-verbal behaviours as well as the words you use when conversations on the topic pop up. Dr Timothy Sharp recommends 'Get comfortable with it yourself, explain your circumstances to those you want to as best you can, when and where you want, and for others, try to not worry it. The most important thing is you and your happiness and health and wellbeing within the relationship, and if other people don't get it, well sometimes they won't – you can't please all the people all the time.'

Sleeping separately, and being open about the fact that you do, is about confidence in your decision, confidence in the reasons for your separate beds, and confidence in yourself and your partner.

PAUSE FOR THOUGHT...

- How do you feel about telling others of your choice to sleep separately or have some type of alternative sleeping arrangement?
- Do you feel confident about your decision and do you think this confidence will come through if you were to speak about your separate sleeping?
- Do you have, or do you need to develop strategies to cope with negative reactions from other people?
- How do you react when other people speak about their sleeping arrangements? Are you aware of how you react?
- What facts do you have prepared if you are not openly comfortable talking about your arrangements, but find yourself in a situation where you don't have a choice?

⑧
Night night, sleep tight

Towards the end of 2012, and in the midst of writing this book, I went with a friend to see the movie *Hope Springs*, hoping to have a bit of a light-hearted laugh at an unashamedly middle-aged girly flick. However, as the opening scene unfolded my eyes rolled in my head with dismay. Meryl Streep's character readies herself in a bathroom and then appears in the bedroom of her husband, played by Tommy Lee Jones. Immediately we know it's HIS bedroom, not theirs. Her romantic overtures are rebuffed by her husband and she retreats to her bedroom, licking her emotional wounds. Again, her bedroom is very obviously the main room that used to be theirs. The movie epitomised every cliché of what separate rooms can signify for a couple. It screamed, 'You are in separate rooms because your marriage has failed'.

I was tempted to jump up in the cinema and shout to everyone, 'It doesn't have to be this way. Sleeping in separate rooms does NOT mean your marriage is over', but I thought I would save my friend the embarrassment. For those who have not seen the movie, it traces the attempts of a couple in their fifties to reinvigorate their failing marriage. The film relies on every cliché about what can go wrong in a marriage between an older couple – lapsed communication, no sex life to speak of, ill-fitting and dull clothing, and an over-reliance on each other and television to fill their lives. It really epitomised for me everything that can go wrong in a relationship – if the couple chooses to let that happen.

The reality is that every couple, whether dating or married, together for a short while or a lifetime, has the choice to make their relationship what they want it be. Not what the movies, the television, their family or their friends say it should be. This is the main message of this book.

You define your relationship, and you determine what is good for you and what isn't.

- Sleeping apart does not mean your relationship is falling apart.
- Sleeping apart does not mean your relationship will fall apart.
- Sleeping apart from your partner does not define your relationship.

Sleeping in the same bed every night won't save a troubled relationship. I don't deny that sharing a bed is the cornerstone of some people's relationship and the glue that helps them stick together, but it is not everyone's glue.

I've said it before and I'll say it again – relationships are tough. Every relationship is tough, and the closer we become to a person, the more likely that person is to see all the bad bits of us and vice versa, which is what creates the hard work. But we also know that good things come from hard work.

Much of the advice provided in this book could be used to approach a range of relationship issues. The core messages of the advice are work hard to have strong, honest communication with your partner and respect each other. These are neither new nor revolutionary ideas, but fundamental skills needed to make any relationship work.

As far as my relationship with my husband is concerned, I do know that we are missing out on something by not sharing a bed every night. But this is just the same as we are missing out on something because we don't get up and exercise together every morning, or have a dedicated date night with each other, or fervently support a football team together. However, there are lots of other 'somethings' that we have in our relationship that other couples don't have.

Fraser and I simply cannot sleep together. Love each other dearly, but can't sleep together. We're certainly not alone, and I'm definitely not worried about the fact that we don't sleep together because I've now met so many happy, healthy couples – some together for nearly 50 years – who don't need to sleep in the same bed every night to keep their relationship on track. So I know that we aren't alone or unusual in our decision to have separate rooms.

All the couples I interviewed were asked how sleeping separately had impacted on their relationship and if given the chance, would they change their current arrangements. The majority of them would like to be sleeping together, but know they can't, so they are happy with their current arrangements. Others, however, don't wish to change their current arrangements because they enjoy the benefits of sleeping alone while knowing they have a successful and happy relationship.

I'm happy at where we're at now. We have flexibility to sleep together or apart and don't need a more formal arrangement.
Ann, married 19 years

Given a choice we would keep the same arrangement – the way we have it now. We recently talked about moving the new baby

into a room of her own and I suggested Doug's room. Straight away he said 'no' and that we would build downstairs before that would happen.
Penny and Doug, married 14 years

It would be great to be able to sleep in the same bed every night, definitely. But we've decided that this arrangement is just better. I get a good night's sleep, she gets a good night sleep. Everything's cool. We still love each other. There's no problem.
Matt, married 20 years

The simple fact is we have a lot of sleep incompatibilities so we both like having the freedom of our own beds and rooms. We're very happy to have separate rooms, but we do both like that our rooms are connected. It gives us a togetherness.
Richard and Catherine, married 20 years

We're happy with the current arrangements. We get along better because there's no resentment because we are sleeping better. Life works better when at least one of us is well rested. I couldn't imagine life with both of us sleep deprived.
Suzette, married 17 years

It's just a different version of normal.
Brooke, married 30 years

We're past thinking that we are missing out on anything. You think when you get married or move in with another person that they are going to be the last person you see at night and the first one in the morning. After realising there were some big problems about all the bits in the middle, we got over that rapidly. I'm happy with the current arrangement. It's what's kept us together.
Caroline, married 7 years

Having felt like I was trapped for so long, I feel like I own something for the first time. I own my own space. This is mine. I can decorate it how I want and be in it how I want. Now that I see it can work I don't think it's odd anymore. I think it will keep us sane.
    Anne, married 20 years

I don't feel that we are missing out on anything. I think we are gaining a fresher outlook each day. I don't think I'm losing anything and as long as my husband is open and honest with me and lets me know he's not losing out on anything, then I will be happy.
    Charlotte, married 1 year

We have an inseparable bond that isn't affected at all by sleeping in separate rooms. We're like two old oak trees planted next to other, and our branches are growing together entwined as we get old together.
    John, married 30 years

The constant evolution of human relationships assures us that what was unthinkable twenty years ago is now not only thinkable but probably in practice in contemporary society. My generation has seen divorce become socially acceptable, defacto relationships become as valid as marriage and same-sex relationships commonplace and almost mainstream. How and where a couple arranges to sleep should be afforded the social generosity given to other behaviours that push the boundaries of what a couple 'should do'.

    I cannot know if sleeping separately speaks of issues that go beyond your need to have a good night of uninterrupted sleep. That is your personal domain. What I can tell you is that as part of a happy and healthy relationship, sleeping in a separate bed every night, or just some nights, means little. Done well it should help a happy and healthy environment flourish because both people feel valued, heard and respected. And they are getting great sleep to keep them functioning.

When you feel confident and comfortable about what you are doing, that infiltrates all that you say about it to others. You don't have to advertise your personal decisions, but nor should you feel embarrassed about making such a practical decision. It's just sleeping at night – no-one's going to lose an eye or a limb over the decision.

So go forth and sleep apart, don't fall apart.

Night, night.

Author notes

Page 4 '**Social dictates as to how a person sleeps ...**' Dittami, J., Keckeis, M., Machatschke, I., Katina, S., Zeithlhore., Kloesch, G., 'Sex differences in the reactions to sleeping in pairs versus sleeping alone in humans', *Sleep and Biological Rhythms*, vol. 5, no. 4, pp 271

Page 4 '**... sleep customs may not always be in the health interests...**' Dittami, J., Keckeis, M., Machatschke, I., Katina, S., Zeithlhore., Kloesch, G., 'Sex differences in the reactions to sleeping in pairs versus sleeping alone in humans', *Sleep and Biological Rhythms*, vol. 5, no. 4, pp 272

Page 5 '**Sleep, as well as being a process, is also a behaviour ...**' Klosch, G., with Dittami, J., and Zeitlhofer, J. *Sleeping better together*, Hunter House Inc., Canada, 2011, p2

Page 5 '**Paul Rosenblatt, professor of family social science at the University of Minnesota ...**' Rosenblatt, P. C., *Two in a Bed: The Social System of Couple Bed Sharing*, State University of New York Press, NY, 2006, p13

Page 5 '**We find the idea strange as society has conditioned us ...**' <http://today.ninemsn.com.au/article.aspx?id=7947365>

Page 5 '**It represents this cookie-cutter model ...**' <http://www.washingtonpost.com/wp-dyn/content/article/2006/01/09/AR2006010901549.html >

Page 6 '**According to most television trivia sources ...**' <http://www.funfactz.com/tv-facts/the-first-couple-to-be-shown-in-bed-1734.html>

Page 6 '**Other trivia buffs claim ...**' <http://www.snopes.com/radiotv/tv/marykay.asp>

Page 7 '**CBS suggested that the beds be ...**' <http://www.imdb.com/title/tt0043208/trivia>

Page 8 '**Couples today are writing their own script ...**' <http://www.spaceandculture.org/2007/03/15/rewriting-marriage-two-beds-bedrooms-at-a-time/>

Page 8 '**A survey by the National Sleep Foundation in 2001 ...**' <http://www.huffingtonpost.com/josey-vogels/couples-sleep-separately_b_1212775.html>

Page 8 '**Studies in England ...**' <http://www.dailymail.co.uk/home/you/article-475998/Why-bed-hopping-save-marriage.html>

Page 8 '**Gopal Ahluwalia, of America's National Association ...**' <http://www.guardian.co.uk/world/2007/mar/12/usa.richardluscombe>

Page 9 '**Sleeping either in groups ...**' Klosch, G., with Dittami, J., and Zeitlhofer, J. *Sleeping better together*, Hunter House Inc., Canada, 2011, p5

Page 10 '**This practice is identified in writings ...**' Klosch, G., with Dittami, J., and Zeitlhofer, J. *Sleeping better together*, Hunter House Inc., Canada, 2011, p34

Page 10 '**The understanding from writings of ...**' Klosch, G., with Dittami, J., and Zeitlhofer, J. *Sleeping better together*, Hunter House Inc., Canada, 2011, p35

Page 11 '**He says that "sensible Victorians ...**' <http://women.timesonline.co.uk/tol/life_and_style/women/relationships/article6008921.ece>

Page 13 '**How each individual ...**' <http://www.sciencenews.org/sn_arcpp/9_25_99/bob2.htm>

Page 13 '**Despite being at an age when their libidos ...**' <http://www.mynippon.com/romance/married.htm>

Page 13 '**Walking marriages reflect sweeping changes ...**' <http://en.wikipedia.org/wiki/Marriage>

Page 14 '**While there do not appear ...**' Klosch, G., with Dittami, J., and Zeitlhofer, J. *Sleeping better together*, Hunter House Inc., Canada, 2011, p74

Page 15 '**Among Orthodox Jews, ...**'<http://www.jewfaq.org/sex.htm>

Page 15 '**The Koran instructs Muslim couples ...**' <http://www.islamswomen.com/marriage/fiqh_of_marriage_9.php>; <http://quod.lib.umich.edu/k/koran/ (4:34)>

Page 16 **'The Queen of England and Prince Phillip ...'** Sally Bedell Smith, 'Love and Majesty', *Vanity Fair*, January 2012. Available online at: <http://www.vanityfair.com/society/2012/01/queen-elizabeth-201201>

Page 16 **'And it's not just royalty ...'** <http://ohnotheydidnt.livejournal.com/70070135.html>

Page 16 **'American designer Diane von Furstenberg ...'** <http://www.thesundaytimes.co.uk/sto/style/living/relationships/article158684.ece>

Page 17 **'A seemingly more successful couple ...'** <http://www.helena-world.com/>

Page 17 **'In a paper considering if sleep was an activity worthy of sociological consideration ...'** Taylor, B., 'Unconsciousness and Society: The Sociology of Sleep', *International Journal of Politics, Culture and Society*, 1993; vol. 6, no. 3, pp 463–471

Page 21 **'Without any question or doubt ...'** <http://plato.stanford.edu/entries/alcmaeon/>

Page 21 **'Positive effects of sleep ...'** <http://www.better-sleep-better-life.com/benefits-of-sleep.html>; <http://longevity.about.com/od/lifelongenergy/tp/healthy_sleep.htm>

Page 22 **'A lack of sleep has serious effects ...'** <http://www.uptodate.com/contents/classification-of-sleep-disorders>

Page 22 **'Klosch reports that while studies find only minor ...'** Dittami, J., Keckeis, M., Machatschke, I., Katina, S., Zeithlhore., Kloesch, G., 'Sex differences in the reactions to sleeping in pairs versus sleeping alone in humans', *Sleep and Biological Rhythms*, vol. 5, no. 4, pp 271–276

Page 22 **'Klösch reports that while studies ...'** Klosch, G., with Dittami, J., and Zeitlhofer, J. *sleeping better together*, Hunter House Inc., Canada, 2011, p35

Page 23 **'When it came to the perceived effects ...'** 'Health Supplement', *The Weekend Australian*, 16–17 June 2012, p 5

Page 23 **'Klösch explains that because of biological ...'** Klosch, G., with Dittami, J., and Zeitlhofer, J. *sleeping better together*, Hunter House Inc., Canada, 2011, p75

Page 23 **'A 2012 study by the Appleton Institute at the Central Queensland University ...'** <http://www.sealysleepcensus.com.au/docs/SleepCensusFinalReportApril2012.pdf>

Page 24 '**Of these, 43 per cent believed ...**' <http://www.sleepfoundation.org/article/press-release/annual-sleep-america-poll-exploring-connections-communications-technology-use->
Page 25 '**In fact, an Australian study in 1997 ...**' <http://www.anzca.edu.au/resources/professional-documents/documents/professional-standards/professional-standards-43.html>
Page 26 '**Bob Ellis, an Australian writer ...**' <http://www.abc.net.au/unleashed/167376.html >
Page 27 '**Sleep deprivation leads to ...**' <http://www.apa.org/topics/sleep/why.aspx?item=1>
Page 27 '**On the issue of weight alone, ...**' <http://health.howstuffworks.com/mental-health/sleep/basics/sleep-obesity.htm>
Page 28 '**A 2010 study at the Woolcock Institute ...**' <http://www.abc.net.au/catalyst/stories/2987827.htm>
Page 29 '**Klösch speaks of historical writings in China ...**'
Klosch, G., with Dittami, J., and Zeitlhofer, J. *Sleeping better together*, Hunter House Inc., Canada, 2011, p39
Page 30 '**Researchers at the University of California, San Francisco ...**' <http://www.ucsf.edu/news/2009/08/4281/first-human-gene-implicated-regulating-length-human-sleep>
Page 30 '**Common consensus from sleep researchers ...**' <http://www.sleepfoundation.org/article/how-sleep-works/how-much-sleep-do-we-really-need>
Page 30 '**A different suggestion by Neil Stanley ...**'
<http://womenworld.org/health/why-you-don-t-need-8-hours--sleep.aspx>
Page 30 '**And another view is offered by historian Roger Ekirch ...**' <http://www.bbc.co.uk/news/magazine-16964783>
Page 30 '**The Division of Sleep Medicine at Harvard Medical School ...**' <https://sleep.med.harvard.edu/>
Page 30 '**The National Institute of Health in America ...**' <http://www.helpguide.org/life/sleeping.htm>
Page 32 '**Research suggests that four to five sleep cycles ...**'
<http://healthysleep.med.harvard.edu/healthy/science/what/sleep-patterns-rem-nrem>
Page 33 '**A 2011 study supported by the National Institute of Health ...**' <http://www.aasmnet.org/articles.aspx?id=2307>

Page 33 '**A 2009 study by the American Academy of Sleep Medicine** ...' <http://www.aasmnet.org/articles.aspx?id=1320>

Page 33 '**In 2012** ***The Weekend Australian*** **newspaper reported the findings** ...', 'Health Supplement', *The Weekend Australian*, 16-17 June 2012, p 5

Page 39 '**The 2012 study by the Central Queensland University** ...' <http://www.sealysleepcensus.com.au/docs/SleepCensusFinalReportApril2012.pdf>

Page 40 '**I find shared sleeping**...' *The Weekend Australian*, Jan 21-22, 2012.

Page 42 '**Paul Rosenblatt, author of** ***Two in Bed: the Social System of Couple Bed Sharing*** ...' Rosenblatt, P. C., *Two in a Bed: The Social System of Couple Bed Sharing*, State University of New York Press, NY, 2006

Page 43 '**And while there are behaviours and habits** ...' <http://www.ncbi.nlm.nih.gov/pubmed/10918859>

Page 43 '**Even though Paul Rosenblatt** ...' Rosenblatt, P. C., *Two in a Bed: The Social System of Couple Bed Sharing*, State University of New York Press, NY, 2006, p13

Page 44 '***Persons most at risk*** ...' <www.sleepfoundation.org>

Page 45 '**The average snorer emits a noise level** ...' <http://www.dailymail.co.uk/news/article-1220595/Meet-grandmother-snores-111-decibels--louder-JET-plane.html>

Page 46 '**This is equivalent to the** ... ' <http://www.industrialnoisecontrol.com/comparative-noise-examples.htm>

Page 46 '***The Guinness Book of Records*** **reports** ...' <http://www.powells.com/biblio?show=0553587129&page=excerpt>

Page 46 '**This puts her as just a little louder** ...' <http://hearing-protection.4ursafety.com/articles.html>

Page 46 '**As a guide, anything over 70 decibels** ...' <http://www.industrialnoisecontrol.com/comparative-noise-examples.htm>

Page 46 '**An outlaw who lived in** ...' <http://en.wikipedia.org/wiki/John_Wesley_Hardin>

Page 47 '**We all change sleeping position** ...'<http://www.dailymail.co.uk/health/article-2110674/How-stop-husband-wife-wrecking-nights-sleep-snoring.html>

Page 49 '**One theory is that women** ...' <http://www.thetimes.co.uk/tto/health/article1963959.ece>

Page 49 '**This is backed up by Paul Rosenblatt's research ...**'
Rosenblatt, P. C., *Two in a Bed: The Social System of Couple Bed Sharing*, State University of New York Press, NY, 2006, p65

Page 56 '**The Big Sleep Survey conducted in 2010 in Australia ...**'
<http://www.sleepsurvey.net.au/the-sleep-survey/results/>

Page 56 '**while the Central Queensland University study ...**' <http://www.sealysleepcensus.com.au/docs/SleepCensusFinalReportApril2012.pdf>

Page 57 '**A 2009 study of 21,475 adults ...**' <http://uninews.cqu.edu.au/UniNews/currentEdition.do>

Page 57 '**Having a room of one's own was a revelation ...**' 'Health Supplement', *The Weekend Australian*, 16-17 June 2012, p 5

Page 58 '**Then there are those who can't face eight hours of slumber ...**' <http://archive.supermarketguru.com/page.cfm/30169>

Page 59 '**In 2011, Ikea conducted a study of two million people ...**' <http://www.apa.org/topics/sleep/why.aspx?item=1>

Page 59 '**Almost a third of participants ...**'
<http://www.sleepsurvey.net.au/the-sleep-survey/results/>

Page 59 '**... the Central Queensland University study reported 77.9 per cent of respondents ...**'
<http://www.sealysleepcensus.com.au/docs/SleepCensusFinalReportApril2012.pdf>

Page 60 '**If this is the area that troubles you most ...**' <http://www.sleepfoundation.org/sites/default/files/sleepinamericapoll/SIAP_2011_Summary_of_Findings.pdf>

Page 61 '**Scientists that conducted the study found ...**' <http://www.dailymail.co.uk/sciencetech/article-2178090/Too-light-night-causes-depression.html>

Page 69 '**Some interesting facts to leave you with from ...**'
<http://www.sleepfoundation.org/article/sleep-america-polls/2005-adult-sleep-habits-and-styles>

Page 88 '**Douglas Stone, Bruce Patton and Sheila Heen's book ...**' Stone, D., Patton, B., & Heen, S., *Difficult Conversations: How to Discuss What Matters Most*, Penguin Books, New York, NY, 2010

Page 90 '**Thomas Bradbury and Benjamin Karney ...**' Bradbury, T., Karney, B. *Intimate Relationships*, Norton W. W. & Company Inc, New York, NY 2010

Page 99 **'Tina B Tessina, an American psychotherapist points out ... '** <http://www.ehow.com/feature_12158549_two-beds-better-one.html>

Page 100 **'Dr Neil Stanley points out that, 'We are the only species ...'** http://www.dailymail.co.uk/femail/article-1303935/More-couples-opting-separate-bedrooms--surprising-results.html

Page 101 **'Stanley makes the point ...'** <http://www.independent.ie/lifestyle/independent-woman/health-fitness/is-sleeping-the-new-sex-1766358.html>

Page 101 **'She also challenges the assumption ...'** <http://www.harpyness.com/2011/01/31/on-living-together-but-sleeping-separately/>

Page 101 **'Klösch describes the association of ...'** Klosch, G., with Dittami, J., and Zeitlhofer, J. *Sleeping better together,* Hunter House Inc., Canada, 2011, p52

Page 103 **'In discussing this issue in her book *A Strange Stirring* ...'** Coontz, S., *A Strange Stirring: The Feminine Mystique and American Women at the Dawn of the 1960s,* Basic Books, New York, NY, 2011

Page 110 **'In their article 'Giving Up and Giving In: ...'** Impett, E.A., Gable S.L., & Peplau L.A., 'Giving up and giving in: the costs and benefits of daily sacrifice in intimate relationships', *Journal of personality and social psychology,* 2005: vol. 89, no. 3, pp 327-44

Page 110 **'This type of sacrifice moves ...'** Gable, S. L., 'Approach and Avoidance Social Motives and Goals', *Journal of Personality,* 2006; vol. 74, pp 175–222

Page 120 **'In his book *Consensus* ...'** Dressler, L., *Consensus Through Conversation: How to Achieve High-Commitment Decisions,* Berrett-Koehler Publishers, San Fransisco, 2006

Page 123 **'John Gottman, psychologist and researcher who runs *The Love* ...'** <http://www.gottman.com/49847/The-Love-Lab.html>

Page 130 **'Klösch says that 'sleeping as a pair is not ...'** Klosch, G., with Dittami, J., and Zeitlhofer, J. *Sleeping better together,* Hunter House Inc., Canada, 2011, p122

Page 135 **'That said, extreme temperatures in sleeping environments ...'** <http://healthysleep.med.harvard.edu/healthy/science/how/external-factors>

Page 138 'This story from the *Wall Street Journal* may provide ...' <http://online.wsj.com/article/SB20001424052748703846604575447380187007528.html>

Page 148 **'Dr Timothy Sharp, Clinical and Coaching Psychologist ...'** <http://www.thehappinessinstitute.com/>

Page 149, **'Dr Barbara Bartlik ...'** <http://bottomlinepublications.com/content/drafts/sleep-apart-grow-closer/print?tmpl=component>

Page 151 **'Stephanie Coontz, director of public education for the Council of Contemporary Families in Chicago ...'** <http://www.quotationspage.com/quote/1990.html>

Page 169 **'Maslow's ...'** <http://en.wikipedia.org/wiki/Maslow's_hierarchy_of_needs>

Page 173 **'A 2007 article from the *New York Times* ...** ' <http://www.nytimes.com/2007/03/11/us/11separate.html?_r=2&oref=slogin&>

Page 192 **'Klösch notes that 'Separate bedrooms are becoming ...'** Klosch, G., with Dittami, J., and Zeitlhofer, J. *Sleeping better together,* Hunter House Inc., Canada, 2011, p144

Acknowledgements

In writing this book a number of people supported me and I would like to thank them.

Jill (especially), Anna and Gordon shared a welcomed candour and an endless willingness to give of their time to question my thoughts and words, and often offer me some better ones. Karen, Kim and Sandra also wielded red pens and friend-grown honesty when called upon to do so. Mum and Stazza reacted to each development of the process with a boundless enthusiasm that always brought a smile to my face.

The encouragement I received from so many other family members and friends was always welcomed and often gave me a needed boost. While the list is long and I thank everyone for their genuine interest and encouragement, I would like to note: Richard, Vicki, Lauri, Brett, Albert, Peter E, Belinda, Jayne, Sarah, Maria, Moyra, Sandy, Holly, Jules, Jane, Steve, Phil, Cindy, Ian, Bern, Julie, Wendy, Chris, Jo, Fraser2, Bernadette, Lesley, Brian, Lisa, Kerri, Peter S, Dan and Bev.

This book was borne of a discussion with a friend and fellow separate sleeper, Sue. I thank her for her early input into the project and her thoughts and conversations shared so willingly.

I would to particularly thank all the people who shared their stories with me. With such a personal subject, the willingness of strangers and friends to share was most appreciated.